EXTINCTION REBELLION

FIGHT with FACTS

Dr. Bob O'Connor

Total Health Publications

2020

DEDICATION

--To the thousands of scientists who have warned us about the dangers of
climate change, and those working for solutions,
--To Al Gore who vividly brought it to our attention,
--To Greta Thunberg who is today the leader of the people who want change NOW.

RECENT BOOKS BY DR. O'CONNOR

Make America Great Again—Like Norway

Abortion—Dissecting the Old and NEW Arguments

Abortion is Good for America and the World
    —Why the Opposition--

Revitalizing Democracy—After Trump, Brexit and Bush

LOVE—The You, The Me, The Us

Extinction Revolution—Fight with Facts

> ➢ Intelligent people know that global warming causes climate change.
> ➢ Intelligent people know that people are the major reason.
> ➢ Intelligent people know that greenhouse gases cause it.
> ➢ Intelligent people know that people are already sick and dying from it.
> ➢ Intelligent people know that we may be too late to save our home.
> ➢ What they may not know is that there are many greenhouse gases.

What they may not know is that overpopulation is the major cause, as more people use more fossil fuels and eat more methane producing animals and fruits and vegetables that used N_2O producing fertilizers. They move to cities built on fertile soil and move into and work in concrete buildings that emitted a great deal of CO_2 in their production.

> ➢ What they may not have thought about is that fossil fuel producing and using industries have the backing of the governments their finances have put in office.
> ➢ Reducing overpopulation will be fought by some powerful religions and by reactionary forces in society that back the long-held traditions.

But the essential changes can be made through the democratic process—however they will be major inconveniences for all—citizens, legislators and businesses.

ARE YOU STILL INTERESTED IN MAKING THE PLANET HABITABLE?

TABLE OF CONTENTS

CHAPTER 1
WHY NOT BURY YOUR HEAD IN THE SAND?

Why the Extinction Rebellion? British politicians realize that Brexit is more important than addressing our path to extinction. The American President, Donald Trump, knows there is no climate change. The thousand thermometers around the world, that have measured global temperatures for the last 100 years, are wrong— because today's American economy is more important.

Intelligent and informed people all know that climate change is seriously threatening our human race, our planet, and our ecological neighbors--both animal and vegetable. We know about:

THE HOT--SNOWBALL EFFECT

➢ More people in our overpopulated world use more fossil fuels and produce more greenhouse gases

➢ These gases warm the air and increase water vapor

➢ This heats the air even more since water vapor is a greenhouse gas

- Less arable land
- More famines
- More forest fires
- More violent storms as upper air cools—releasing the water vapor as rain and snow
- Oceans warm and become more acidic—reducing shellfish
- Permafrost thaws releasing more methane
- Ground-level heat and air pollution sicken and kill millions

➢ Air and ocean warm more—glaciers and Arctic and Antarctic ice sheets melt

- Sea levels rise-- less living area and less farmland for a growing population
- Under-sea reservoirs of CO_2 and methane are released
- River transportation of goods severely reduced due to reduction of glacier volume
- Less fresh water due to glacier melting (higher costs for desalinization)
- Water wars—migration wars

➢ Severely reduced population survives in the far north and far south of the hemispheres

BUT WHY WORRY? SOME HOMO SAPIENS MAY SURVIVE!

THE MENTIONED AND UNMENTIONED CAUSES

Technology, based on fossil fuel use, is the obvious cause of global warming and climate change. The resulting cause is greenhouse gases from fossil fuels-- the hidden cause is overpopulation.

We expect our politicians to create laws to force a reduction of greenhouse gases. We expect scientists to aid in this effort. But to reduce population???
- I want children.
- It is a God-given right and obligation.
- We need more consumers for the things we produce.
- We need more soldiers to protect us from: the Russians, the Americans, the Chinese, and the Lilliputians!

And does overpopulation create other social problems? YES!

So let's look at all the issues, from fossil fuels and technology to overpopulation--and suggest some possible solutions.

If we want to slow these effects--controlling climate change depends on reducing greenhouse gases and increasing sinks--like vegetation. We have practically used up our major sink—our oceans.

The higher the income, the more CO_2 is produced because of the amenities of money: driving, air conditioning, consuming food requiring more energy to produce, living in bigger houses (energy cost of building materials), air travel, etc.

WE MUST NOT CONFUSE WEATHER AND CLIMATE

Weather is the day to day experience of heat, rain and other factors of nature that we will encounter over a short period of time, like a day, week, or month. Climate is the long-term averages of weather—usually a term of at least 25 years.

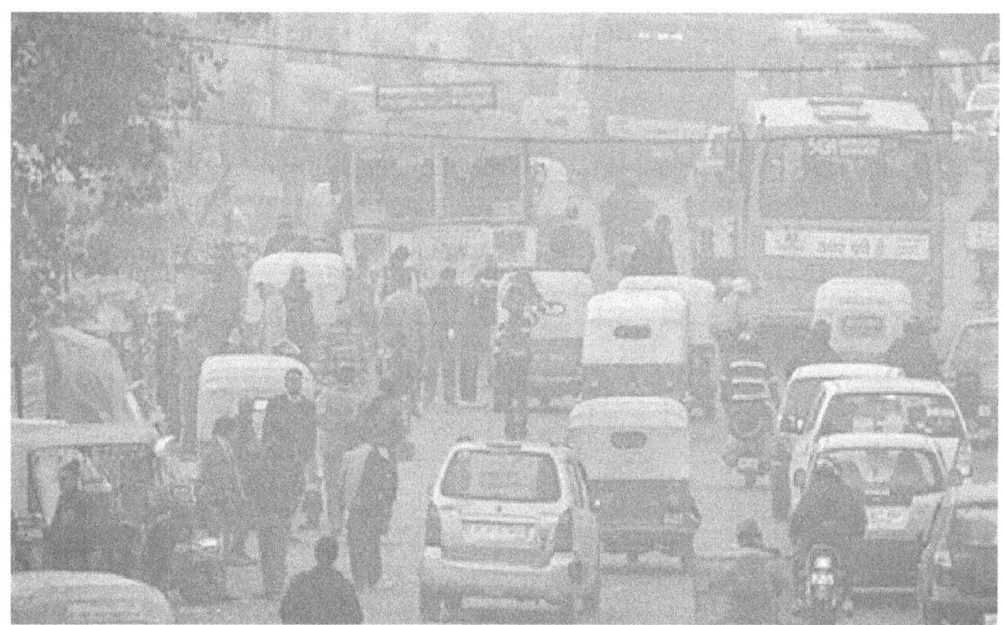

HOW DOES IT HAPPEN?

Briefly, this what happens. The sun emits rays (photons or waves), in a broad spectrum of wavelengths. From less than a billionth of a meter to over 1000 meters. We can see only a small part of the spectrum—waves that are 2.5 to 5 millionths of a meter (about 60 to 120 thousandths of an inch). Ya! Really teeny!

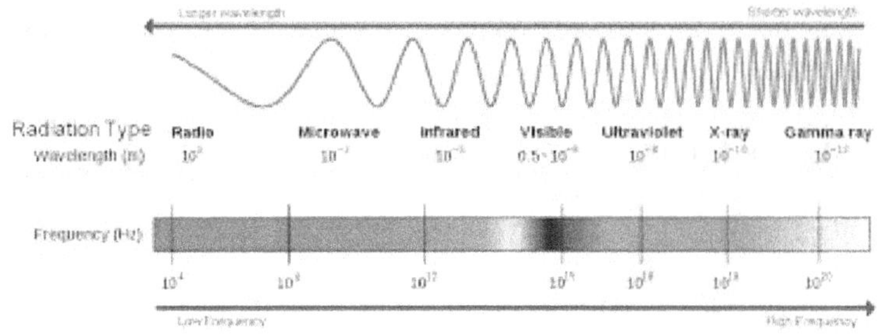

What we think of as heat waves are in the infra-red area of the spectrum. When you go to the beach on a sunny day, much of the heat you feel is infra-red, most of the tanning comes from the ultra-violet rays. But all rays can heat a surface. You have probably cooked in a microwave oven. The waves are 1 to 10 centimeters (1/2 to 4 inches). And you may have heard of cancer patients being burned when treated with x-rays. This seldom happens now because doctors are aware of the correct dosage. Microwaves are longer than we can see, and x-rays are shorter than we can see.

WHAT ABOUT THE SKEPTICS?

Global warming skeptics often argue that the rise in temperatures is a phenomenon of nature like the warm period from about 800 to 1200 AD or the little Ice Age, from about 1300 to 1850. But these were geographically limited areas that were affected. Today the temperature change affects the whole planet. Skeptics may argue that it is a result of a shifting polar vortex--a low pressure cold area near the poles. They generally don't think that carbon dioxide can cause it all. But coring into the deep Antarctic ice, yielding 800,000 years of climatic evidence, shows no rapid increase in temperature like we see today. And the burning of fossil fuels during the last 270 years gives us a strong case to explain the rapid rise in the world's temperature.

History   of   global   surface   temperature   since

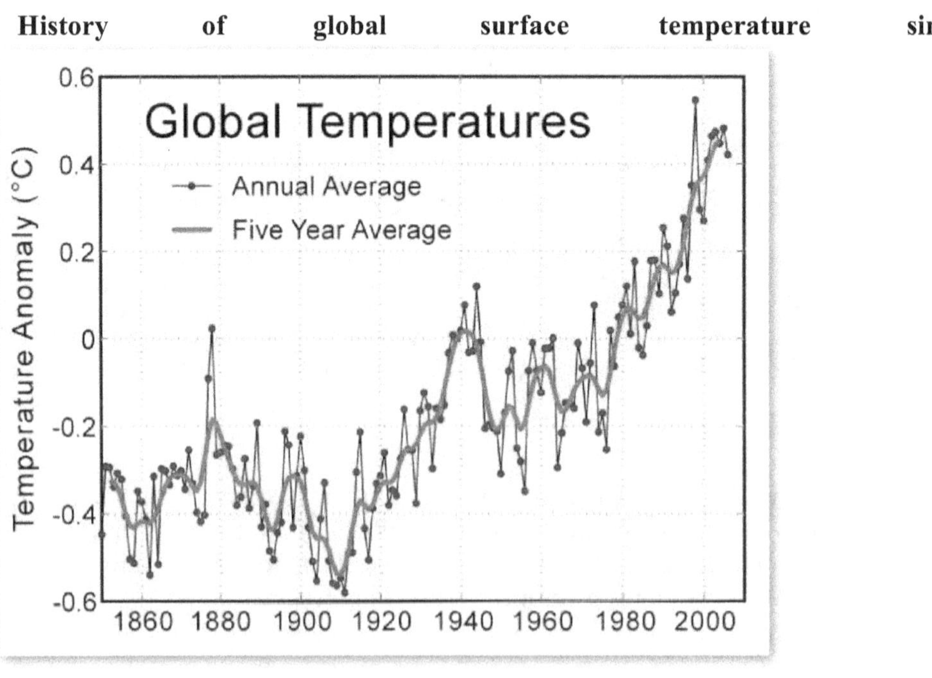

1850

THE PROPAGANDA OF THE SKEPTICS' ARGUMENTS

Propaganda attempts to influence people to a particular point of view using techniques to cloud the issue or deflect arguments. We see this in politics all the time. In the climate change issue, industries that might be hurt if climate change politics legalized the major methods for controlling CO_2 or methane emissions. What if no more coal or oil were allowed to be extracted from the bowels of the earth, or all cattle were required to be killed to reduce methane production. You would certainly expect the coal and oil industries to mount a propaganda offensive—an d they have! What about the cattlemen and the dairy farmers? They have, too—but to a much lesser degree. But, as you understand, there is more money in oil than in steaks!

It seems that whenever a person or a group wants something bad enough, they will do whatever is necessary to make it happen—but you say, "That's not m or al!" But it has value from a self-centered value assumption. (The other assumptions that we might use are: God-based assumptions or society–based assumptions.) The great philosopher Immanuel Kant wrote that: we should always treat people as ends in themselves, not as means to our own desires. Most people who study ethics think that this should be our prime value for the treatment of others. But people, or special interest groups, disregard this standard and do whatever is necessary to get what they want.

While we generally say that we prefer honesty in our leaders, his tor y—particularly recent his tor y—shows that lies and rationalizations can change how, or if, we vote. George W. Bush's campaign allied with a group that called his opponent, John Kerry, a coward and a traitor. None in the group had ever served with Kerry, who had served in combat in Vietnam—where he was awarded three Purple Heart medals for injuries and a Bronze Star for bravery. About ten years later, the group revealed that it was all a lie. Bush had avoided the war by serving in the Texas National Guard, where he did not follow some important orders.

In the Brexit vote in the UK in 2016, those who wanted to leave the European Union outfitted a bus with signs that indicated that the British were paying 350 million pounds a week to the European Union and that the money could be sent to the National Health Service (NHS) to improve British health care. It was widely publicized and changed many votes. But it was all untrue.

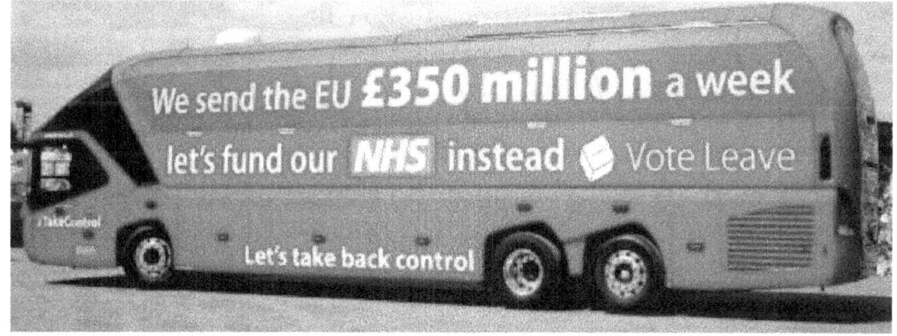

The day after the election the perpetrators of the propaganda admitted that no money would have gone to the NHS. Also, the actual fact is that the UK really paid only about 250 million pounds a week to the EU after a rebate negotiated by Margaret Thatcher. Then the UK has money returned from the dues for farm subsidies, research and other income. The actual contribution was 117 million pounds a week much of which went for government administration and contributions to East European countries to help their economies so that they will become more lucrative trading partners eventually.

In the 2016 American election debates Donald Trump promised to eliminate the national debt in 8 years. But he has added $3.1 trillion to it in less than three years—with a strong economy.

Barack Obama focused his campaigns on "hope." Some was realized, some was not.

Mitch McConnell, majority leader of the Senate, disagreed with the impeachment vote against Trump and gave a long speech against impeachment. He gave many reasons, historical and philosophical. Along with some truths, there were some lies. For example, he mentioned that it took only months (3 months from the time of the wh is tleblower's charging that the President had withheld military aid from Ukraine unless he would investigate Joe Biden, a possible presidential opponent, and his son). Actually, it was about five months. It took three months from the official charges to the impeachment. McConnell said that it took years of investigation of President Clinton before he was impeached. Actually, it took eleven months from his perjury to his impeachment.

We are all familiar with the term "fake news." We are bombarded with it— an d many people believe it.

The point is that we are lied to continually in many areas of our lives. Industries have much to lose in the short term, and they have millions of dollars to develop and circulate false or incomplete information in their propaganda. They fund non-pr of it "think tank s" with funds that are not taxed because they are giving to non-pr of it or ganizations-- that they control.

Nearly two hundred arguments have been used, usually violating the official rules of logic. For example, there are many studies that have charted earlier climate and earth temperatures. Some have studied tree rings, some have analyzed ice cores or sediment cores. One that I recently heard was an economist criticizing one of the tree ring studies that deduced that the temperature of the reg ion-- in which the trees grew 500 years ago—was criticized because it was in a limited area of the world. He then concluded that global warming was not happening.

A few of the commonly used arguments are:
➢   The climate has changed before
➢   The sun is causing the temperature change
➢   There is no consensus that it is happening
➢   It's not as bad as the climate scientists say it is
➢   The records are not reliable

But, 97% of scientists studying the climate say that the danger is severe and we humans are causing it. The sun can be a minor factor, but fossil fuels are the major cause. There has never been a climate situation like this, barring the occasional excessive cooling from volcano clouds or the crashing of a giant meteorite.

The scientists use over 1,000 thermometers on land and sea that have been used for between 50 and 100 years. The skeptics don't seem to have even one thermometer and they don't have records for the last 100 years that they can compare with those of the climate scientists.

The truth is that the advertisers and propagandists are smarter than we are. In order to see through the lies and rationalizations, we must have a far better knowledge of math, science, and logic. The 2018 international education testing (PISA—Programme for International Student Assessment) indicates that the UK is down the list—an d the U.S. is even farther down.

PISA rankings 2018
SCIENCE

Rank Country Score
1   China   590
4   Estonia   530
8   Canada   518
14   UK   505
18   US   502

MATH
Rank Country Score
1   China   591
8   Estonia   523
12   Canada   512
18   UK   502
37   US   478

WHY ARE WE SO OFTEN CONVINCED BY FAKE NEWS AND OTHER PROPAGANDA?

Is it our inferior knowledge of the facts, as shown in the low PISA scores? The United States is 37th internationally in math and 18th in science for 15 year-olds? The U.S, spends more money on education than any of the countries that perform better. Why are we uneducated? (See "Revitatizing Democracy" by the author to understand the problems in American education—and some solutions.)

> Is it that we trust our elected representatives even if they are indebted to special interests?
> Is it our very high level of adult illiteracy? 32 million US adults can't read.
> Of those who can read, 72% have read a book this year—mainly fiction.
> Of the young (18 to 28) about 10% watch national and international TV news
> Of those with a high school education about 30% (all ages) watch TV news.

So where do Americans get their information? From one source?, like: the usually reactionary and conservative Fox News, the liberal and moderate CNN, or the foreign sources of international news like BBC or Al Jezeera. If people are to participate in their democracy effectively, they must see all sides of the issue, have enough knowledge of history and science to understand the situation, and have enough of a grasp of the tools of logic to see any fallacies elucidated by: the news outlets, advertisers, politicians, and propagandists.

One major type of logical fallacy is criticizing an idea because one, or some, who hold the idea are criminals. This is called the *ad hominem* fallacy. One such use of this propaganda was that "The Unabomber believes in climate change." (The Unabomber is a mathematical genius who was one of Harvard's youngest graduates and the youngest mathematics professor ever hired at the University of California. He came to believe that industry was ruining human life, so he decided that by killing some people he could gain attention to his belief.) His belief in climate change has nothing to do with his criminal behavior!

Another approach is to appeal to our emotions rather than our intellects. None of us want climate change to be true. But unfortunately, it is true. So giving people a false hope that it may not be true is emotionally warming, but the warmth disappears under the cold logic of hard facts.

We encounter fake news continually, For example, for a number of years, as the autism spectrum increased significantly, parents had to blame something other than themselves. Their children had been vaccinated against smallpox, measles and some other diseases that earlier had scourged our children. Many parents refused to have their children vaccinated and actively promoted the an ti-vax movement. Then, lo and behold, a measles epidemic erupted in 2019. The number of US cases increased from 86 in 2016, to 120 in 2017, to 375 in 2018, to 1300 in 2019. The World Health Organization reports that there were 140,000 deaths in the world from measles in 2018—the huge majority of which would have been prevented with vaccinations.

If we look to science for an explanation for the autism spectrum occurring, there is no evidence of vaccinations causing it. But there is evidence of both genetic and epigenetic causes. Genetic causes include the passing on of genes that affect and cause autism or genes that may prevent it by allowing for normal neurological development. Epigenetics is a science, initiated about 30 years ago, which looks at how environmental factors can make certain genes work or not work because one or more genes can be compromised by methylation (CH_3). One such gene DLGAP2 (Discs-Large Associated Protein 2) is significantly related to the development of autism.

In a recent study conducted at the Duke University Medical Center, it was found that fathers who had smoked marijuana had this gene methylated. "This gene is involved in transmitting neuron signals in the brain and has been strongly implicated in autism, as well as schizophrenia and post-traumatic stress disorder." (Murphy SK, et al. "Cannabinoid exposure and altered DNA methylation in rat and human sperm." Epigenetics V 13, Issue 12, Dec, 2018. Article available at: (https://www.tandfonline.com/doi/full/10.1080/15592294.2018.1554521)

Another recent study of marijuana smoking mothers showed a large number of health problems with their infants. The effects of cannabis smoking mothers on their children's possible autism was not studied. (Gunn JKL et al. "Prenatal exposure to cannabis and maternal and child health outcomes: a systematic review and meta-analysis." British Journal of Medicine Open, . 2016;6:e009986. Available at: https://bmjopen.bmj.com/content/6/4/e009986?utm_source=TrendMD&utm_medium=cpc &utm_campaign=BMJOp_TrendMD-0S

An earlier study, from 1992, did not involve epigenetic research (the science was in its infancy). It involved pregnant mothers using some form of cocaine. The findings attributed its effects on the children's development in the intrauterine environment, but epigenetic causes may, and probably were, involved. The cocaine use of the pregnant mothers caused "significant neurodevelopmental abnormalities that were observed, including language delay in 94% of the children and an extremely high frequency of autism (11.4%). The high rate of autistic disorders not known to occur in children exposed to alcohol or opiates alone suggests specific cocaine effects." (Davis E et al "Autism and developmental abnormalities in children with perinatal cocaine exposure." Journal of the National Medical Association. 1992 Apr; 84(4) 315-319)

The point is, that people, sincere or insincere, may rationalize, lie or engage in propaganda to convince us of their ideas. We should make sincere and comprehensive scientific investigations to determine the truth or falsity of what we are told. Presidents, priests, politicians, and parents will tell us things that they want us to believe. Their sincerity should not obscure the truth!

CHAPTER 2
PROBLEMS RELATED TO CLIMATE CHANGE

What effects will global warming have on our lives?

The ramifications of global warming are vast. Many species will disappear. That may not be so bad as long as it is flies and mosquitoes, and maybe rattlers, but I hope it's not pandas and porpoises.

SOCIETAL PROBLEMS

MORE DRY LAND AND DROUGHTS

While increased rain and storms will affect parts of the world, increased heat and dryness will affect other parts. Lands affected by drought have doubled since 1970. Southern Europe is predicted to warm considerably as the century stumbles along under the burden of global warming. While we saw temperatures rise significantly in the early years of this century, we also saw the underground water tables dropping as less rain cooled the summer swelter. Forest fires from Portugal to Greece, and in the U.S. and Australia, warned us of the parching earth and drying vegetation, which was becoming less friendly to the farmer.

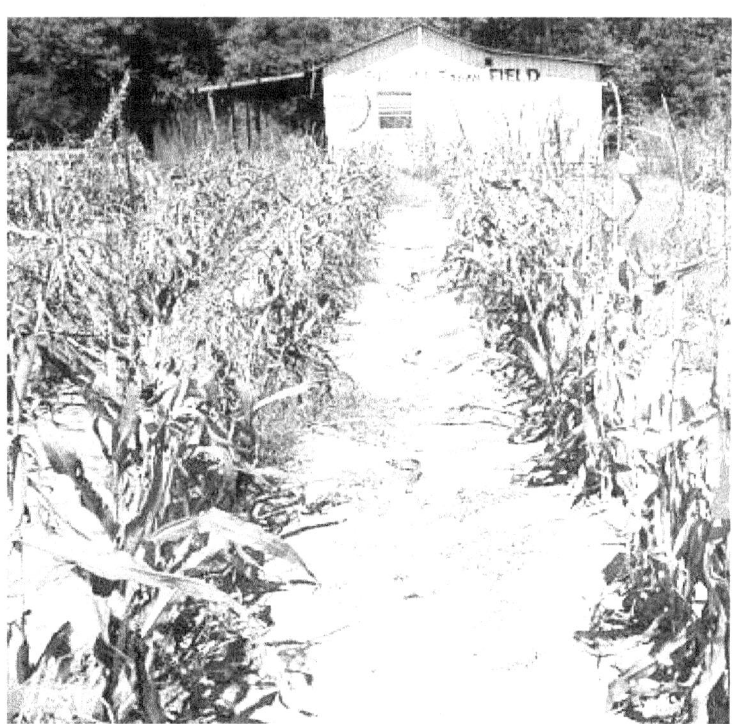

Parched corn

Is the Sahara leaping over the Mediterranean? The mounting evidence is that it is more than a momentary flight of the Fahrenheit—it is the result of the increased global warming. It is the desertification of the fertile lands that gave us the Renaissance, the Age of Discovery, the Age of Enlightenment, and the Industrial Revolution. By century's end

Italy's average temperature is predicted to rise by 8 degrees—ten times the last century's temperature rise. The number of uncomfortably hot days of 35 degrees Celsius, 95 Fahrenheit, should increase tenfold. Rainfall is predicted to drop 15%. Farming will be decimated.

Tourism will drop as people leave the beaches of Spain for those of Denmark and Norway. Emigration from southern Europe will increase and the northern EU countries will be the destinations.

Portugal has experienced severe drought, their worst in history. Crops have died as have their farm animals. Another problem is that as the rivers carry less water, hydroelectric plants cannot put out the electricity of which they are capable.

In China, sub-Saharan Africa, and Kazakhstan the deserts are expanding--sometimes because of poor farming methods and sometimes because of diverting the water that is upstream, which makes the downstream communities waterless. A related problem is that when lakes, rivers and seas dry up, the fish will die. The Aral Sea in central Asia, which once supplied a million pounds of fish yearly, had practically dried up. Thanks to a World Bank loan to Kazakhstan for a dam, the north side of the sea is being filled. The south side, in Uzbekistan it is still dry. Lake Chad, in Africa, once the continent's largest body of water, has been reduced to 5% of its former girth. Diseases like malaria have increased in the higher altitudes, such as in Kenya, which used to be too cold for mosquitoes. There will be more pressure for North Africans to emigrate northward. It's not fair, but the countries that cause most of the global warming are not suffering from it as much as many of the Third World countries.

FOOD SHORTAGES AND FAMINES

As the heat rises and the humidity drops progressively in the areas north and south of the equator, farmland in the temperate zones is becoming less productive. As heat and arid conditions chase the farmers towards the poles, water for irrigation is becoming less plentiful. As the needs of the human and animal populations compete with the needs of industry, farmers often hold the last tickets in the line for water rights. In California's great central valley, on less that 1% of America's farmland, farmers produce 8% of the nation's agricultural production. More than 230 crops are grown, including 60% of the world's supply of almonds. About 16% of the nation's irrigated land is here. In the north, the American River brings water from the Sierra snowpack near lake Tahoe. But in the central and southern parts of the valley, pumped groundwater supplies much of the H_2O. In some areas, so much has been pumped from the ground that the farms are sinking. State authorities forecast eliminating 800 to 1300 square miles of farmland from the state's water supply. What will this do to the agricultural employment sector and to food prices.

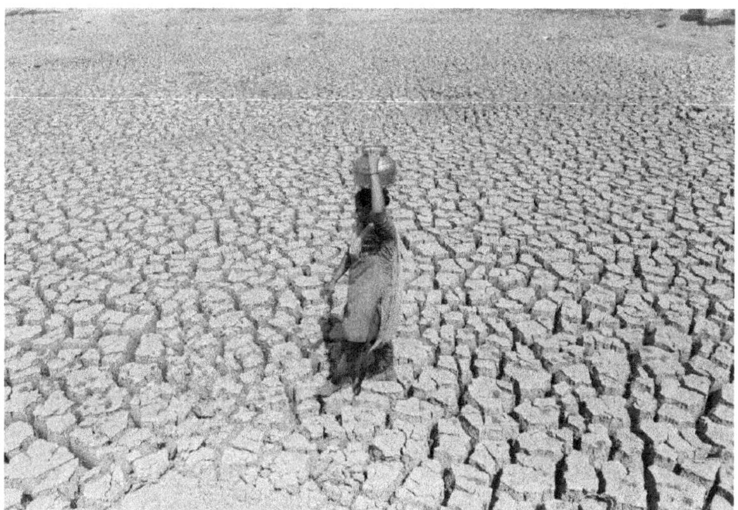
Parched land—Where is the water I need?

Mass extinction has already hurt agriculture. Bats, bees and birds that pollinate plants are down 17%. A United Nations' report estimates that 75% of the world's food crops rely on pollinators to some extent. If these species go extinct, so does almost 8% of the world's food species. A third of the fishing areas are already over-fished. Everyone will be affected in ways that are difficult to imagine now.

FAMINES

Famines in the last 20 years have occurred mainly in sub-Saharan Africa. In Ethiopia, Congo, Sudan, Somalia, Mali, Nigeria, and similar countries. But who cares if millions of people starve to death because of climate change and war, when we are comfortable in our well-nourished air-conditioned northern hemisphere. The Economist has called this the "forever famine." The main hospital in Niger treats hundreds of malnourished children every week. Part of the problem is that there are few dams to store needed water for homes, farms, and herders.

HIGHER OCEANS

18,000 years ago, at the peak of the ice age, the sea level was 120 meters lower than it is today. For the last 3,000 years, the ocean has risen only a foot or two, that's less than a half inch (1 cm) per 100 years. But the predictions now are that warming will raise the sea level over a meter this century. That's more than 3 feet. But, and it's a big 'but', three million years ago when the temperature rose 2 to 3 degrees above today's temperature, the sea level rose by 80 feet, not 3 feet. The ice sheets at that time melted much faster when the temperature changed than we have been predicting today. And you know that the rise in the oceans is caused by both the melting of glaciers and ice sheets that are over land, and the increased volume of the ocean due to its warming—water expands as it warms.

Satellite surveys show that arctic ice is melting faster than we thought it would. Snowfall will increase in the polar areas because of the increased water vapor in the air, but not enough to make up for the loss of ice through the warming of the air and sea.

Scientists predict that by 2050 temperatures will have caught up with today's level of CO_2. That's when there will be no Arctic ice in the summer. The dark ocean that replaces it will absorb even more heat. It will create a chain reaction that will further heat the earth's temperature even if we stop emitting additional greenhouse gases.

This doesn't even consider the worst-case scenario, which has only a 5% chance of happening—that would be a rise of 6 feet in the sea level by 2100—with 1.78 meters (5 feet, 10 inches) of that coming from melting ice sheets and 22 centimeters (nearly 9 inches) from the warming of the oceans.

Researchers tell us that if the rise of greenhouse gases is not stopped, the glacial melting can add as much as 24 feet (7.5 meters) to the level of the oceans in 200 years.

TIDAL FLOODING FROM HIGHER OCEANS

Flooding from the ocean is a combination of the mean water level (caused by glacial ice-melt and the expansion of the ocean because of warming), the high tide, and the size of the waves.

The Union for Concerned Scientists, looked at 52 National Oceanic and Atmospheric Administration tide gauges in coastal cities in Florida, Maryland, Georgia, Virginia and other states. The UCS analyzed the states' flooding risk under mid-range sea level rise predictions taken from the White House's National Climate Assessment — an estimate of 5 inches of sea level rise by 2030, and 11 inches by 2045. It found that tidal flooding could triple in some cities in 15 years and occur 10 times as often in most cities in the next 30 years.

This are not the type of flooding that kills people, but rather the type that does damage to homes and businesses. A rise of 11 inches in the water level by 2045 would increase the high tide by that much. To tell you what this means, if there was a slope of 1 foot per 30 feet of beach, the high tide would reach about 30 feet farther towards the land, in 2045, than it does today. Then combine that with any higher than normal waves and you have a problem. Then, of course, if the waves are much higher because of the storms that global warming often increases, you have a multiple problem.

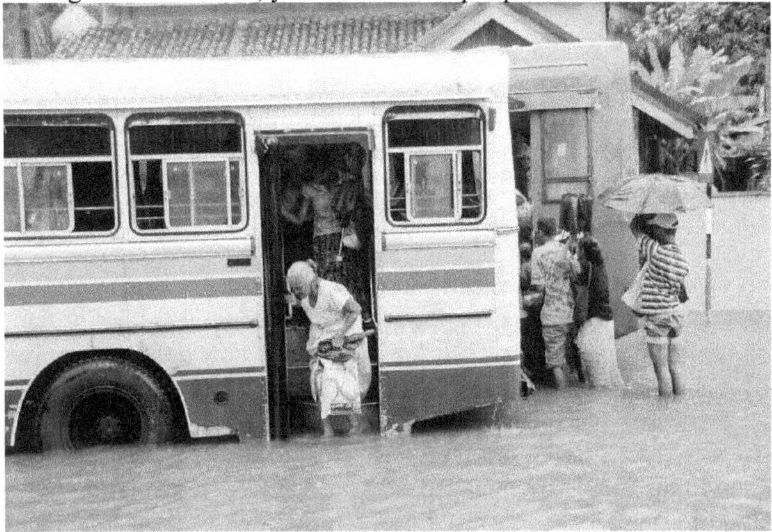

TIDES

If you are not familiar with how tides work, here is a brief description. The sun and the moon pull on the oceans. The moon is more important. As the moon circles around the earth it pulls the water towards it. The water nearest the moon and on the other side of the earth will be in high tides, so we can say that if the moon is at 0° and the other side of the earth is 180°, the water at 90° and 270° would be lower, so low tide. When the sun and moon are in line (either on the same side of the Earth, or at exact opposite sides) the tide is highest because of their combined gravitational pull. There are approximately two high and two low tides in a day.

When I was working my way through college as a beach lifeguard at Venice Beach (Ya! "Baywatch") we always had tide books, the same as the fishermen use, to predict the tides. These books tell us to the minute exactly how high the tide would be. In mid-July we had the highest tides of the year, about 7.2 feet above the mean. If we happened to get big surf at the same time, as sometimes happened, we often got water all the way to the back of the beach in pools and several times the door of my lifeguard tower was beaten in by the surf. Sometimes I had to wade to my tower through the 2 foot deep pools created when the big surf crashed over the berm, where the beach begins sloping towards the sea, then flowed deep into the beach. So the tide just tells how high the water level will be then the size of the waves will indicate how much damage will be felt. Both high waves and a high tide can bring water well past what is normal.

At Venice Beach the difference between the highest and lowest tides of the year were about 8 feet. The average difference in the world is 3 feet (1 meter), but in Anchorage Alaska it can be 40 feet, and at the Bay of Fundy in Canada it can be 53 feet (16 meters).

On November 13, 2019 Venice, Italy experienced one of its highest tides, 7 feet, 4 inches (187 cm) above the mean. 85% of the city was underwater, The mayor reported t hat the damage incurred will cost hundreds of millions of dollars to repair.

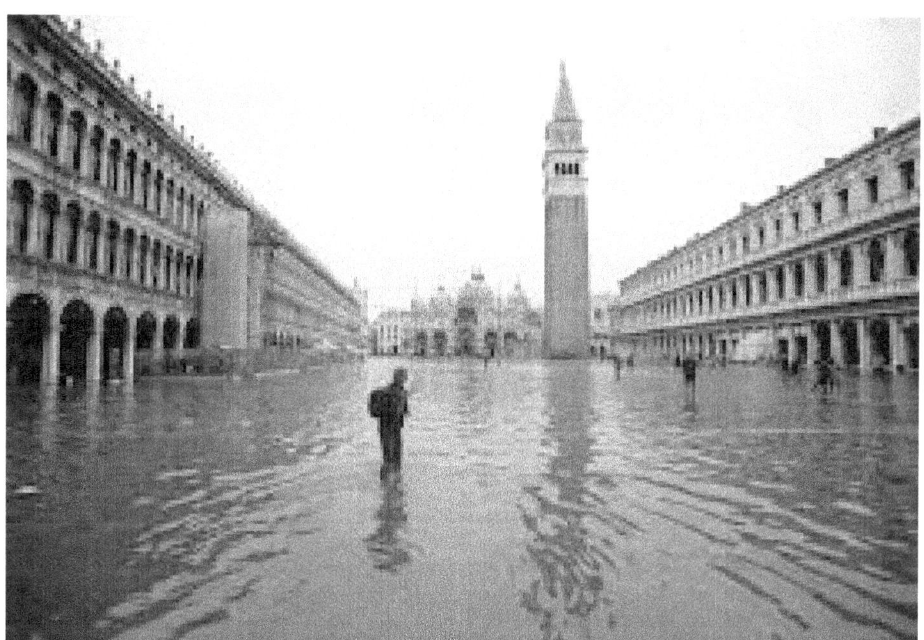

The Doge's Palace and the St. Mark's Cathedral were damaged

WATER LEVEL

The following chart shows how the ocean water level has fluctuated in the last 2000 years. You notice that it goes down during cold periods and up during warm periods. It is far higher today than at any time in the past two millennia.

Reconstructed Temperature

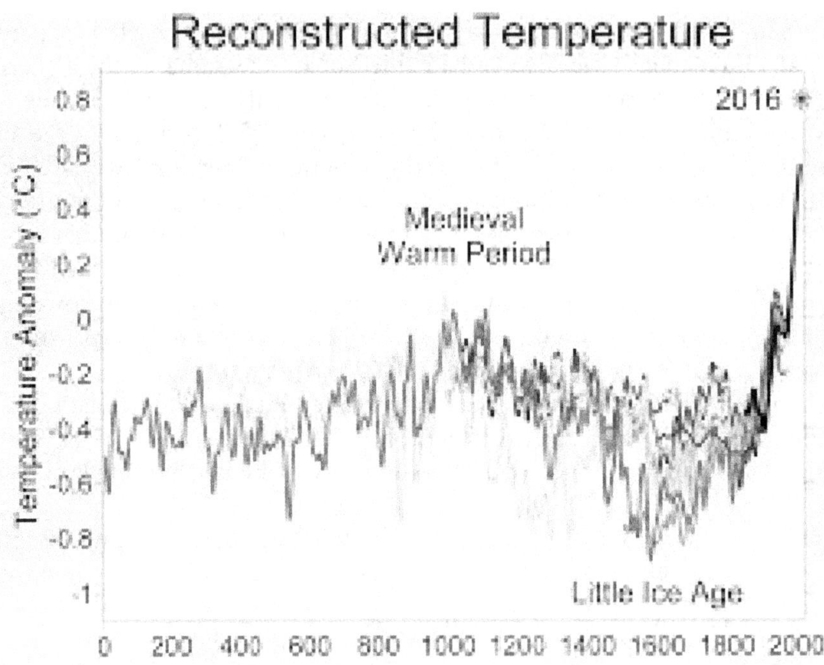

Below is a chart of the last 25 years showing a rise of sea level of nearly 100 millimeters (4 inches). The rise from 1900 to 1990 was between 1.2 and 1.7 millimeters (about 1/20th of an inch) per year. It is now between 3.3 and 4.0 mm per year (about 1/7th to 1/8th of an inch) per year.

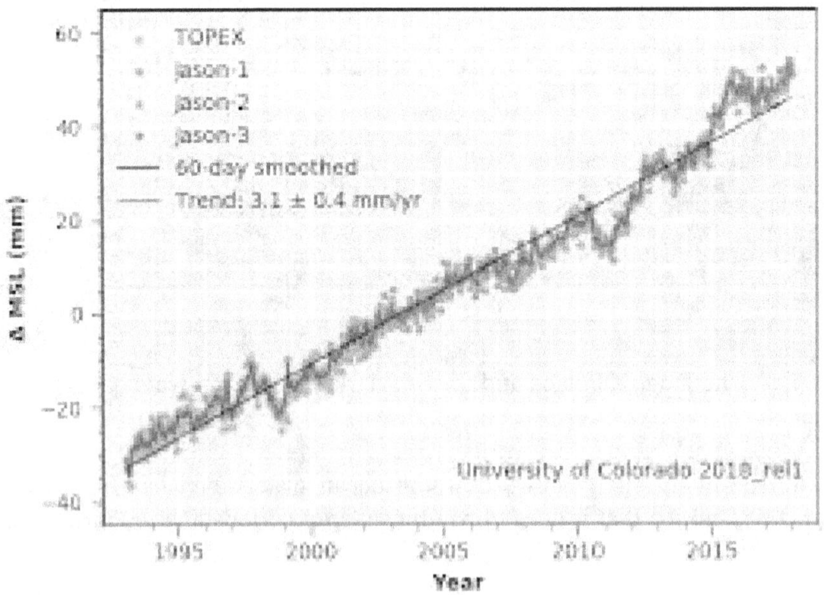

The sea level rise increases in speed as the warmer water expands and as glaciers melt more rapidly.

Since cities are often built by the oceans, because of trade access and more pleasant temperatures, between a half and three-quarters of a billion people (1 in 10 to 1 in 15 people) can be displaced. This would also affect industries near the ocean.

Look at how many cities are built right next to the ocean: New York City, Alexandria, Rio, Shanghai, Norfolk, Boston, Charleston, Miami, San Francisco, Seattle, Baltimore. It has already had a significant impact on the coastal cities of China. Naturally the Netherlands is in real trouble—as is Venice, Italy.

Some of the effects will depend on where you live. Oceans will rise, so coastal living will be destroyed. In less than a hundred years the seas could rise 20 feet, but the projections now are for only a couple of feet. But even this could wipe out costal living from Bangladesh to Malibu. Venice, Italy already has severe problems. And the Netherlands will have to build their dikes much higher, but it's doubtful that the country can survive without periscopes. They'll have to raise seaweed rather than tulips, and cod rather than cows!

High water level caused problems are already evident in some Pacific islands where the inhabitants have had to be relocated because the island was submerging. It has also been true in northeast China where the ocean has encroached on the low-lying land near the ocean. Where this happens, it also makes the ground incapable of growing food because the saltwater changes the chemical makeup of the topsoil.

MORE ACIDIC OCEANS

When you understand that almost 94% of the warming gases have gone into the oceans you can see how it can affect our seas and sea life. So far only about 2.4% percent have gone into the atmosphere. That has warmed our land about 2.1%, and the ice sheets have absorbed the rest – – Arctic sea ice has absorbed 0.8%, the Greenland ice sheet has absorbed 0.9%, Antarctica about 0.2% and the rest by other glaciers. I wonder just how much more the ocean can handle when the percentage of CO_2 will rise past that 2.1 level. Just look at the havoc that 2.1 level has had on droughts, floods, hurricanes and water evaporation.

Along with more water, the CO_2 absorbed in the water has made the surface water 30% more acidic than it was in the pre-industrial age. Acids, like the weak carbonic acid, H_2CO_3, comes from water vapor (H_2O) and CO_2, nitric acid comes from the nitrogen compounds, and the strong sulfuric acid H_2SO_4 is formed by water and sulfur oxides. The sulfur comes primarily from coal burning. The absorption of the greenhouse gases by the ocean reduces the amount of global warming at a cost of increased ocean acidity. But the oceans should be a bit alkaline. The acidity is reducing the ocean animals' abilities to form shells and coral reefs. It is also bleaching the coral—as shown in these photos of the Great Barrier Reef in Australia. The top photo shows how it was some years ago, the bottom photo shows how it was two years ago.

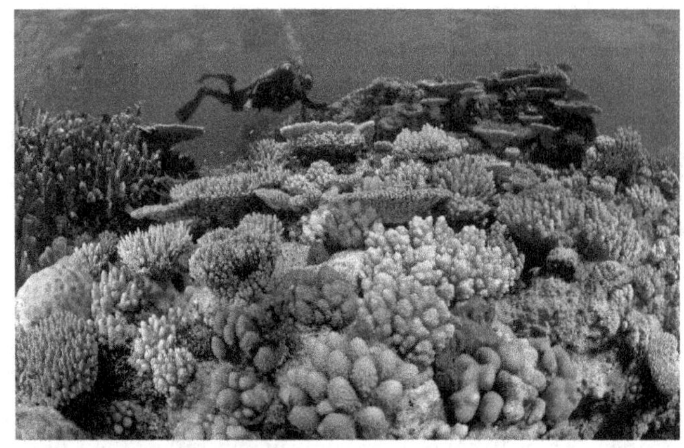

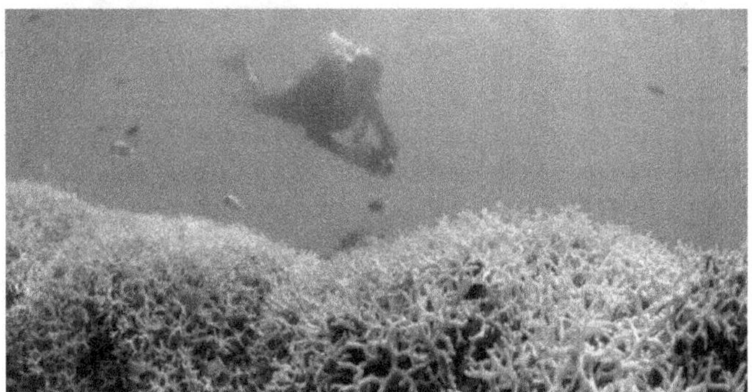

Well over a third of China has been dampened by acid rain from the 25 million tons of sulfur dioxide emitted from their coal and oil burning factories. The Chinese output of sulfur dioxides is increasing almost 10% per year. While the cheaper energy sources are good for business they harm the soil and the vegetation. Sulfur dioxide is not a greenhouse gas but it is certainly an air pollutant. But it's not only China. The eastern U.S. and eastern Europe have also had problems.

At the current level fish are not generally affected but their eggs may well be. Also as the lower-level animals like brittle stars are reduced there is less food for sea mammals like seals. So by affecting lower level sea life, the food chain can be disrupted severely.

STRONGER STORMS

The stronger hurricanes and storms will decimate large areas. This has recently been shown in Puerto Rico and the Bahamas. The stronger hurricanes are, of course, the result of extra water vapor being absorbed into the atmosphere, then dropped on the land through storms. This increases the number of famines where the water had been evaporated and destruction of the areas where the storms hit.

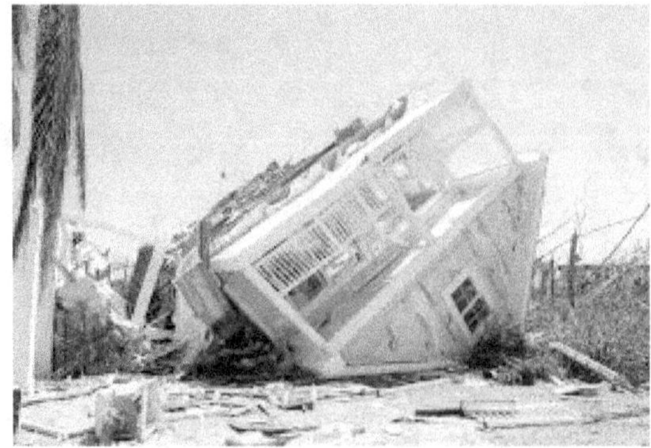

A result of the 2018 hurricane in Bermuda

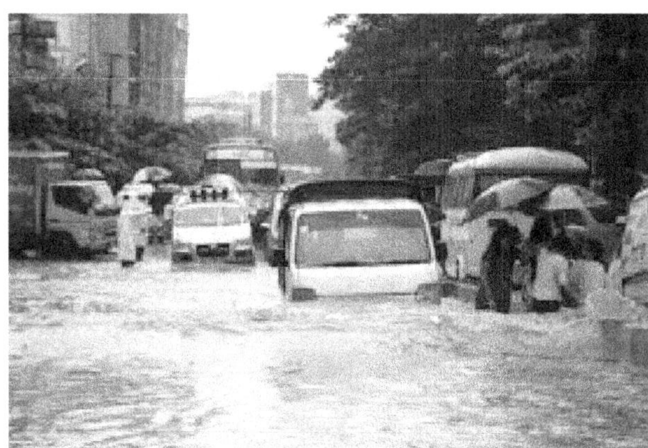
Rainstorm-caused flooding

Droughts and flooding will damage large areas of the earth. Texas has experienced some of this, as have several European countries.

Wind storms can also blow topsoil from farm lands away—often ending in oceans, rivers and lakes.

INCREASE IN THE NUMBER AND INTENSITY OF FOREST FIRES

But people are not the only contributors to the accumulation of greenhouse gases. Nature does its part! Often, we work together to destroy our planet. Our human contributions include drying the air and vegetation so that forest fires are more easily increased in number and severity, In California, sparking wires from power companies have started the fires. In

Brazilian farmers and miners have started the fires to expose the land for their economic desires. For centuries farmers have used fires to nourish their lands.

Records show that in warmer years you can almost always expect more forest fires. Estimates of carbon dioxide emissions from forest fires are as high as 20% of the total. And, with the trees and other vegetation being destroyed, there are fewer carbon sinks to capture the CO_2 in the atmosphere.

And there are life and property dangers. In 2018 the forest fires in Greece killed 91 people. Those in Spain and Portugal killed 70. In the U.S. an average of about 12 people per year are killed in forest fires.

Nearly 23,000 buildings were lost in the California wildfires of 2018. But expenses for fires go well beyond the losses incurred.

More than 140 forest fires in Australia are burning as I write on January of 2020. More than two dozen people have lost their lives, more than 2000 homes have been destroyed—and millions of animals have died. Insurers have already receive claims of over $165 million. (Up go the premiums!) One estimate is that it is costing Sydney businesses $50 million per day because of the smoke, transportation disruptions, and smoke related illnesses. But Australians should breathe a sigh of relief because their prime minister has told them that there is no connection between climate change and the forest fires! But we wonder if he was correct in reversing the actions taken by the previous government to combat climate change. He must have been right because he was democratically elected— and the people know who is best to lead them!

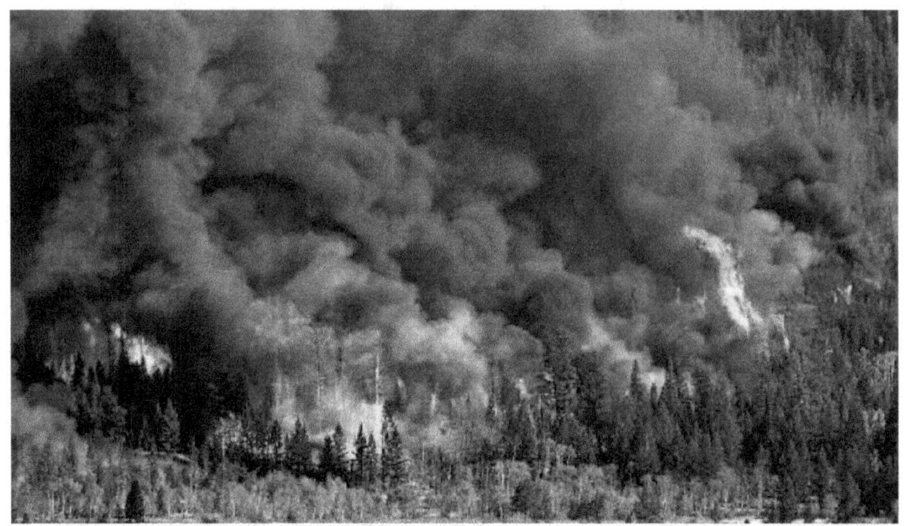

Costs of forest fires are difficult to pinpoint and they vary considerably from year to year. As an example, for 2014, the last year for which total figures are available, we find a loss of $328.5 billion—1.9% of the year's total economic output (GDP). This is broken down into: expenses $273.1 billion and losses from the fires $55.4 billion. Building construction is 17.5% of the total ($57.4 billion). So the preparation to prevent and fight the fires is a large, but hidden, expense.

FOOD AND MEAT PRODUCTION

Rice production contributes about 12% of the methane, and grass or grain eating meat, such as cattle, add another 5%. The increased desire for meat in the richer countries increases the methane production and its absorption into the atmosphere. Approximately one to 1.4 billion cows exist on the planet. They each produce between 70 and 120 kilograms of methane per year. So that is about a trillion kilograms or 1.1 billion tons.

One way that greenhouse gases are often measured is in carbon dioxide equivalents—considering the long-term greenhouse effect. Here are some CO_2 kilogram equivalents relative to producing one kilogram (2.2 pounds) of:

> Beef 18 to 34.6 depending on the country (U.S. is lower, Brazil and Japan are higher)
> Lamb 17.4
> Pork 6.35
> Chicken 4.57

Different studies include different variables. The variables may include: CO_2, methane, manure, cost of slaughter, transportation, electricity used, loss of CO_2 absorption from the grass consumed, food grain factors, etc.

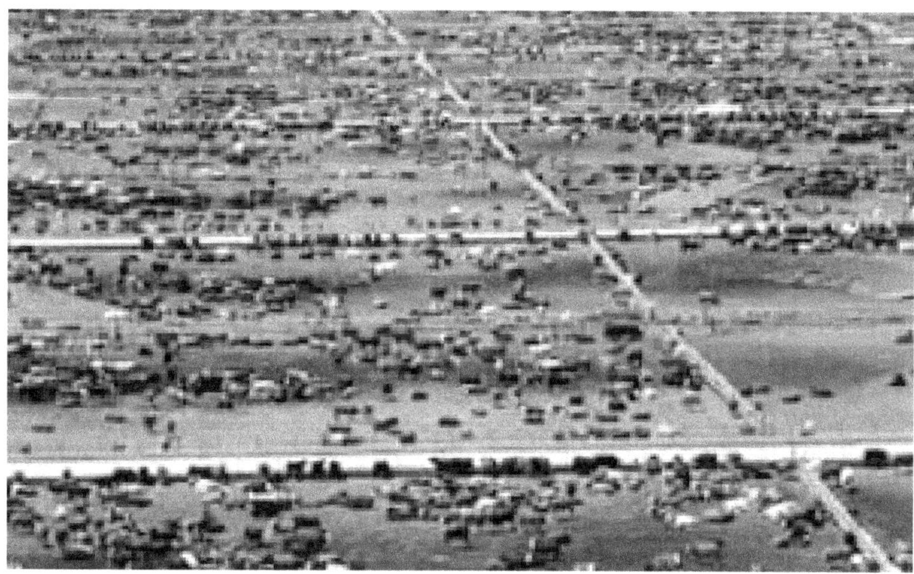

An extensive cattle farm

As electric cars and trucks are produced to fight climate change, oil industry jobs will be lost. As self-driving cars and trucks are developed, the need for truck and taxi drivers will be significantly reduced.

While reductions in coal mining and oil refining may decrease employment in some regions, possibly more people will be employed in the areas of: solar power, hydroelectric power, tidal power, and wind power.

Climate change caused migration has already begun. As heat and flooding continue to make life unsustainable and unbearable, climate migration will continue. In 80 years it is estimated that one in seven people worldwide will become environmental migrants. Other estimates put it at twice that number. According to the United Nations High Commission on Refugees, an estimated 22 million people have been displaced since 2008 because of extreme weather. By 2050 that number is expected to be 700 million.

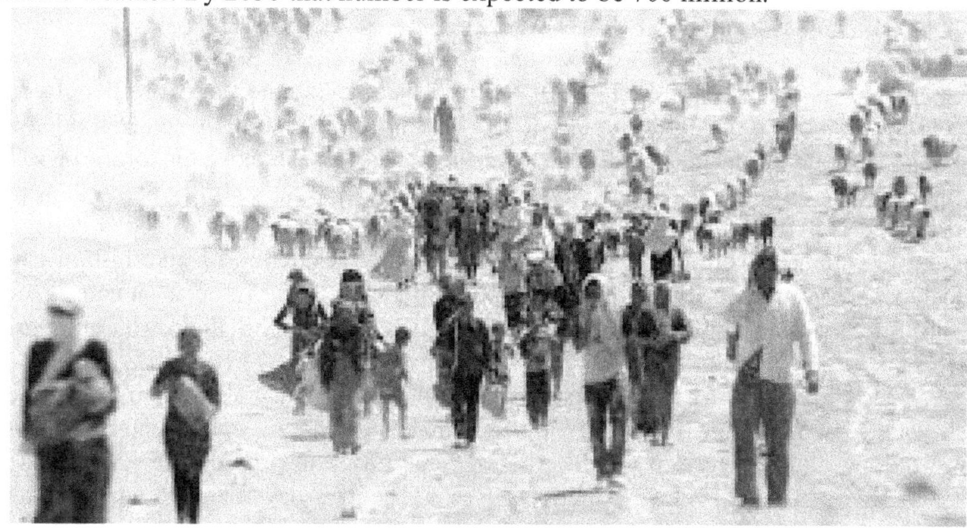

The World Bank estimates that nearly one and a half million people will head to the United States because of climate change in the next 30 years. The World Food

Program reported that nearly half of Central America emigrants left because of food scarcities.

This immigration is likely to meet heavy resistance in the U.S. and the E.U. The economic immigrants and the refugees of the various wars (Iraq, Syria, Yemen, Afghanistan) have tested the empathy and the economic costs of many of the accepting countries.

PERSONAL ISSUES
PERSONAL FINANCIAL COSTS

There will be huge economic effects. Insurance premiums will rise because there will be more forest fires and more hurricanes and cyclones. The risk of natural disasters has more than tripled in the last fifty years. Over a third of these have been climate related. The $15 billion a year increase in insurance payouts has to be covered by increased premiums for fire and flood insurance. More deaths occur during heat spells. This will affect health-insurance premiums. National security will be affected because people will be forced to migrate from parched lands and eventually from submerged lands.

People in hurricane zones will have more and stronger storms. People inland from warmer oceans can expect more tornadoes and much more rain and flooding, such as we have seen in China, Pakistan, India and Europe. People in north and east Africa and southern Europe can expect less rainfall and hotter temperatures, so their agricultural output will drop. In Africa, this will lead to more famines. Africa's population, growing at about 7% a year, will be hard-hit by droughts. Warming and the lack of water will force migration north. And if the will of Allah or God decrees, northern hemisphere countries will allow for immigration. But the immigrants will bring with them their traditions of family fecundity and the white nations will grey as they continue their socialistic support of siring babies. We need only look at Darfur to see the conflict caused by the desertification of large areas causing migration. We already have increasing numbers of global warming refugees to add to those fleeing violence. Then there will be the reduction in income from tourism around the Mediterranean because of too much heat and too little water.

Taxes will increase to pay for the damage done to cities flooded, wind damaged through hurricanes and cyclones, or fire-damaged through forest fires.

Food costs may rise as much farmland is rendered too dry for crops, as winds blow away topsoil, and as available water dwindles.

WATER SUPPLIES

There is not enough fresh water today to supply our needs. More people on the planet require more water to drink, bathe, and cook with. They require more food-- which needs water to be produced. Just about everything we need takes water to produce. Even biofuel, made from corn or switch grass uses between 290 and 2100 gallons of water to produce and deliver a gallon of the fuel. (The large variation of water needed depends on the area in which it is produced,) With today's annual production of nine billion gallons, which is expected to rise, some are questioning biofuels' relative value as an energy aid.

Fire retardants used in fighting forest fires are finding their way into ground water—and severely polluting it.

Desalinization of ocean water is a possible answer to the problem of the lack of fresh water. It costs about fifty cents to a dollar to desalinate a cubic meter of seawater. Using the one dollar figure, it would cost 38 cents a day to provide the 92 gallons (378 liters) of water that the average American uses, 19 cents a day for the average European (22 gallons/189 liters), and 6 cents a day for the average African to use 6.5 gallons (57 liters). Some countries are totally dependent on desalinized water, others are largely dependent on it.

SOME POSITIVES

But there are some positives. Because of Arctic warming, the Northwest Passage will open up and both reduce the shipping costs and the CO_2 emissions from ships going between Europe and Asia. The supertankers that now must travel south of South America, because they are too big for the Panama Canal, will save huge amounts of money in fuel and will be able to make more trips during the summer months.

Russia may also gain as Siberia warms. It may open vast areas for agriculture. But then the planet will lose as the Siberian peat bogs release the carbon and methane that they have sequestered since the last ice age.

But we could replace the energy of all the world's power plants if we could just use effective solar collectors in a small area of the Sahara. An area the size of Portugal would probably do it.

YOUR PERSONAL HEALTH AND CONVENIENCE

Your body temperature is about 98.6 degrees Fahrenheit. At around 104 degrees, organ damage can begin. You can imagine the damage. Heat can kill people directly and indirectly. On May 28, 2019 Turbat, Pakistan recorded a temperature of 129.2 degrees F (54 C)—and I understand that not a lot of people have air conditioning there! In July of 2019, in Phoenix, Arizona it was 112 F (44.4 C) . Not a record for Phoenix—but they have air conditioning. The highest temperature recorded in the UK was in Faversham, Kent, on August 10, 2003. It was 48 C (118.4 F) High temperatures have been recorded in the last 100 years at various places, but not nearly as often as they are today, with the whole Earth and its oceans warming at levels never before experienced in such a short time period.

In October of 2019 in the Sacramento area of California, a seven-day rolling blackout was done to inspect the power company's electrical transmission lines—they had been found responsible for one of the major forest fires the year before. Other California power companies followed suit. More than a million people were affected. So you may not be able to count on electrical power for your AC in times of extreme heat.

Heat can raise people's blood pressure leading to heart disease deaths. Heat waves can therefore raise death rates. One in 2003 in Paris killed 4,870 people, and one in 2010 in Moscow killed 10,860. A recent study in New England found that a one degree Celsius raise in the summer temperature increased the death rate by 1%.

Painful kidney stones can increase if people do not increase their hydration because the increased temperatures increase our perspiration. Solid materials, which should be dissolved and passed in the urine can calcify and become solid "stones" that can become painful blockages in the tubes leading from the kidney to the bladder or from the bladder to the ureter.

According to an OECD report in October of 2019, 40 per 100,000 people worldwide have died because of air pollution, the number was 140 per 100,000 in China and India.

COMMUNICABLE DISEASES

The increased length of the summer season and the increased temperature can increase the number of disease-carrying insects, such as mosquitos, ticks, fleas, and flies. The CDC (Center for Disease Control of the U.S.) reports that diseases from bites from these creatures have quadrupled in the last 15 years, to over 100,000. These diseases include: malaria, dengue fever, Lyme disease, birth-defect causing Zika, encephalitis, and yellow fever — and warmer winters may fail to kill off populations of these insects.

Alaska's warming has found a six-fold increase in stings from wasps, yellow jackets, and bees.

Algae-related complaints. Cyanobacteria, or blue-green algae, thrive and bloom in the rising temperatures of bodies of water, from municipal water systems to the Great

Lakes and Florida's Lake Okeechobee. The algae have been linked to digestive, neurological, liver, and dermatological diseases.

ALLERGIE S

Allergy seasons—from ragweed in the fall to tree pollen in the spring—are lengthened because of less frost and earlier blooming. Fungal spores (those outdoors and in moist basements) will most likely thrive, tickling the throats of many.

MORE HURRICANES AND RAIN

Why have we had increased rains, hurricanes and tornadoes? The ocean absorbs most of the heat from the global warming. This heat leads to the increased evaporation of the water. The warmer air can hold more water vapor. But when the air cools at the higher altitudes it can't hold all the excess water. This gives us increased rain inland from the oceans. The northern plains area of the U.S.A. has had heavy rains from water that had been evaporated from the Pacific. And the inland countries of Europe get what was evaporated from the north Atlantic.

The torrential summer rains have inundated central Europe and caused devastating floods. Prague, my favorite city, was partially under water in both 2002 and 2018.

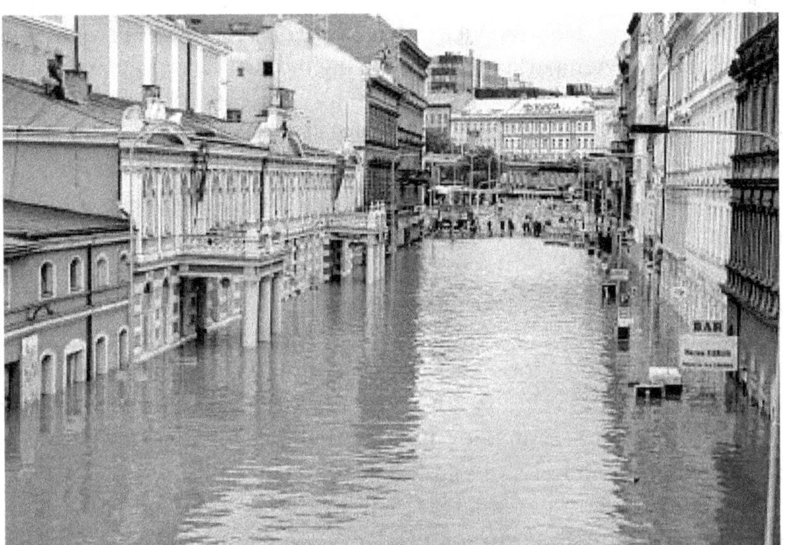

Prague theater during 2018 flood

Floods are normally much more common in the winter from rain and snow melting. There is little doubt that the recent summer floods are caused by global warming.

With warmer oceans, the hurricanes get stronger. The average hurricane has winds 50% stronger today than they had 40 years ago and the number of the strongest hurricanes has doubled. A rise in the world's sea surface temperatures is the primary contributor to the formation of stronger hurricanes. Since 1970 the average temperature of the ocean has risen 0.5 degrees. In the Gulf of Mexico it has risen 3 degrees recently. In the 1970s, the average number of intense Category 4 and 5 hurricanes occurring globally was about 10 per year. Since then it has more than doubled.

Category 4 hurricanes have sustained winds from 131 to 155 mph. Category 5 systems, such as Hurricane Katrina that destroyed New Orleans, had winds of 156 mph or more. Another recent hurricane set a record with winds at 175 mph.

COST OF GLOBAL WARMING TO BUSINESSES AND TO INDIVIDUALS

Insurance costs will go up. Damage costs from the three most expensive types of storms-- hurricanes in the United States, typhoons in Japan, and rainstorms in Europe will nearly double if carbon dioxide emissions double their current rate. If we do nothing, increased hurricanes in the US will increase hurricane insurance premiums to nearly double, to $150 billion. Japanese typhoon costs would nearly double to $34 billion. Flood insurance in Europe will rise significantly to about $150 billion. Fire insurance costs will rise significantly in fire prone areas.

The consumer will pay the costs in increased prices. And, taxes will increase for a number of expenses such as: preventative measures for fire, wind and flood control; aid to victims; low interest loans; and clean up. Fire insurance premiums have risen annually in areas where forest fires are possible. Carbon taxes, where applied, increase the costs of goods. Costs of living due to climate change is definitely increasing!

For businesses, production and transportation will be disrupted. Disruption of workers availability can be due to: storms, flooding, fire, disease, and water shortages. Transportation on many European rivers, such as the Rhine, were diminished, then halted at times in both 2018 and 2019. Severe drought was the major cause. Shipping up-river was disrupted from the port of Rotterdam 760 miles to Switzerland, including the major cities: Cologne, Frankfurt, Dusseldorf, Bonn and Koblenz. These cities are major only because they are on the Rhine River.

The Rhine provides for commercial transportation of industrial goods, for power generation, for power and transportation for industrial production, for drinking water for 25 million people, in addition water for agriculture, the transportation of agricultural produce, and for tourism, including the expensive river cruises. Industrial plants could not get the needed raw materials for their production, nor could they ship them out on the river. When you have 30 million tons of material and goods being shipped from Rotterdam in a year you can understand the problem. If there is not enough water for normal shipping, the barges cannot carry as much tonnage. So more barges are needed—and more fossil fuels to power the additional barges. So the problems caused by global warming require more fossil fuels to solve the problem—then more warming is produced. As often happens, the solution causes more problems.

The Bloomberg chart below indicates the continued drop in water levels at Kaub, a critical are on the Rhine.

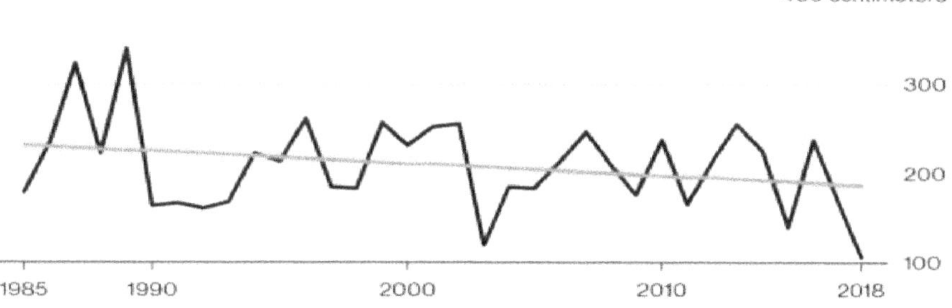

The low water level of the Rhine in the third quarter of 2018 was estimated to have cut German industrial production by 0.8%, or $2.14 billion. (Central Commission on Navigation of the Rhine) Freight rates were raised by both the Rhine and Danube shipping companies because of the low water. You, of course, pay for this in the increased prices of the cars, wine, and other products that use these rivers for transport.

The global warming is melting the glaciers and snowpack faster than normal. Half of the Alps' glaciers are expected to melt within 30 years. This is happening in mountains across the northern hemisphere. This can have major effects on many of the hemisphere's rivers, from the Colorado to the Yangtze.

It has been estimated that if the global temperature rises 2 degrees Celsius (3.6 F) the global economy would suffer a 15% drop, and at 3 degrees C (5.4o F) it would fall 25%, matching the Great Depression of 1929.

1.2 billion jobs are threatened—particularly in fishing, farming and forestry. But jobs in the area of preventing climate change, like solar engineering, could create 24 million jobs.

Nearly 130 military bases of the U.S. Armed Forces, including the Naval Academy, have either suffered damage from climate change or are in imminent danger of being damaged. Because of these and other factors, the U.S. Department of Defense reported in 2017 that climate change is a "direct threat" to U.S. national security. But their Commander-in-Chief, Donald Trump, does not believe it-- because the energy industries, that give him millions of dollars, have told him that climate change and the human causes of it are merely a hoax perpetrated by the Chinese. And if you can't believe capitalist energy billionaires, who CAN you trust???

So while the Earth has been able to handle the natural amounts of carbon in the oceans and on the land, we have added to the problem by going deep into the ground for more sources of carbon in coal, oil and gas –then burned them. We have gone far past what nature can handle. The carbon is here to stay. It is picked up by trees and other plants while they grow, then released when they die. It is picked up in the oceans in plankton and in shellfish then released when they die and decompose. So, the carbon that has always been a part of the life of the Earth-- just re-circulating from air to water to plants to the soil – it is never removed. But the carbon that has been in a long sleep, far below the Earth's surface, has been awakened and threatens us as a malevolent ghost of our evolutionary past. Even if we added more trees to the land and clams to the ocean, we won't be able to exorcise this carbonic ghost.

Maybe we can build a huge exhaust pipe into outer space and get rid of it that way. It's certainly not practical to send one or two thousand rocket ships full of carbon into space every day. We had better find practical solutions fast.

ELECTRICITY GENERATION

Let's look at the major pollution cause, power generation.

On average, about 1400 pounds of CO_2 is created for every million kilowatts of electricity produced. Of course it varies from source to source. The different types of energy sources-- coal, oil, water power, wind, natural gas-- all have quite different polluting effects. Only about 4% of electricity in the U.S. and the world is generated by renewable sources such as wind, solar, geothermal and tidal power. Another 7% comes from water power. You can see from the chart that the percentage of biofuel use is declining somewhat, but it is still at the level of 1990—and that's not good.

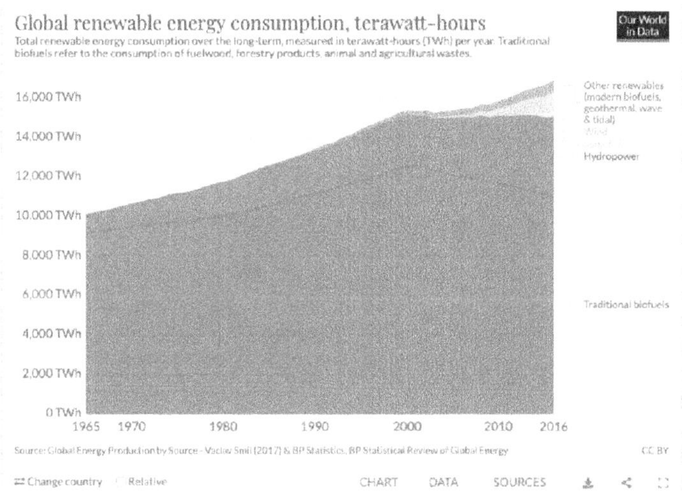

Water power generates only about 7% of the world and US electrical power. Water power generation is, of course, subject to how much rain a watershed gets—and that can vary from year to year. Throughout the world coal, oil and gas provide most of the power for the generation of electricity. They, of course, are the great polluters. With China building nearly 600 coal burning power stations we can expect things to get worse. Although there have been some proposals for building cleaner Chinese power plants, they would be quite expensive.

COAL

The quality of coal is determined by its carbon content. High quality anthracite coal is about 95% carbon and yields about 12,000 British thermal units per pound. Lower grade coals generally contain more than 55% carbon and yield about 7,000 BTUs per pound. In the USA about 27.5% of the energy is produced from coal. All of the sources of U.S. energy are listed below.

As shown in the chart below, oil and coal are still over 60% of our energy sources.

SOURCE	BILLION KILOWATT HOURS	% of TOTAL
Total - all sources	4,171	
Fossil fuels (total)	2,653	63.6%
Natural Gas	1,469	35.2%
Coal	1,146	27.5%
Petroleum (total)	25	0.6%
Petroleum liquids	16	0.4%
Petroelum coke	9	0.2%
Other gases	13	0.3%
Nuclear	807	19.4%
Renewables (total)	703	16.9%
Hydropower	293	7%
Wind	273	6.5%
Biomass (total)	58	1.4%
Wood	41	1.0%
Landfill gas	11	0.3%
Municipal solid waste (biogenic)	7	0.2%
Other biomass waste	-1	<0.1%
Solar	64	1.5%
Photovoltaic	60	1.4%
Solar thermal	4	0.1%
Geothermal	16	0.4%
Pumped storage hydropower[3]	-6	-0.1%
Other sources[3]	13	

With every American using over 12,000 kilowatt hours of electricity each day, that's 440 million kilowatts a year, so you can see the problems. The average American uses about 2 times the energy that the average European uses and ten times what the average Central or South American uses. The American also uses 20 times what the typical Far Eastern person uses and 40 times what the African uses. No wonder the US produces so much CO_2.

There's another source. As mentioned, much carbon is trapped by nature under the permafrost in Russia and Canada. Decayed, but frozen, trees and other vegetation are releasing their stored CO_2. Estimates are that 200 to 800 billion tons of carbon would be released to the atmosphere if the permafrost thaws. So we have a doubly negative effect of our fuel burning. Human yearly output of carbon is 'only' about 7 billion tons of carbon—and look at the mess that has gotten us into. Our increased carbon dioxide in the air warms it so that frozen life in the tundra becomes thawed and releases its carbon. This in turn increases the warming even more. It is estimated that one gigaton of methane will be released in the next 80 years as the permafrost thaws. It is just another illustration that warming increases warming.

Right now, there are more roadblocks than solutions. While any legislator who is not illiterate knows about the global warming problem, they are afraid to address many of the causes of it and would never address our population increase and its negative climate changing effects. But as political pragmatists, they seek to make life sound easier for the electorate. Otherwise they won't get re-elected.

You may have noticed that there is traffic on the roads. All those cars are driven by somebody else's children! Gridlock is the curse of the car. So, the U.S. government plans to spend about $48 billion dollars a year on highways. That should reduce gridlock costs, but it won't if it increases car buying and gasoline usage? And the $48 billion is not enough money to really solve the problems of traffic for 300 million Americans each driving their own car--alone. I read that they would have to spend $70 billion a year to solve the major problems with traffic. After all, the number of vehicle miles traveled has increased by 100% in the last 30 years, but roads have only increased about 10%.

Don't forget commercial trucks that produce about 13% of the CO_2 and they need more roads. Then airplanes add another 4% and that increases yearly.

It's obvious to all that there is too much traffic on the roads. To stop it we must stop people from living modern lives. Would we use our cars if public transportation got us there faster, more comfortably, safer and cheaper? And we should certainly plant more trees.

CHAPTER 3
THE CAUSES OF CLIMATE CHANGE

The world does go through periodic heating and cooling cycles. The skeptics are quite ready to attribute todays temperatures to those multi-millennial planetary causes. So, we will take a quick look at them. But today warming problems are chemical, so we will spend much more time on them.

PLANETARY CAUSES

Our world goes through warming and cooling cycles about every hundred thousand years. We should now be entering a cooling cycle which would've started in about 1970. From 1940 through 1970 our Earth had cooled about 3/10 of a degree Celsius.

The hundred thousand year cycles are divided into approximately 80,000 to 90,000 years of ice age and 10,000 to 20,000 years of warming. Normally the warming comes before the CO_2 is increased. The last 50 years it is CO_2 that is leading the climate change warming.

The last cycle of warmth ended around 10,000 years ago. So we have had a cooling trend since then. This cooling trend would have continued for thousands of years if there were no people. But since 1750 the carbon dioxide content of the atmosphere has deviated from the normal cycle. Instead of the temperature decreasing as expected, it increased because of fossil fuel burning. Methane and nitrous oxide have also increased because of agriculture, with methane being produced by cattle and fertilizer.

The climate change denying politicians have told us that for millions of years the Earth's temperature has risen and reduced. This is true, but what they do not tell us, in fact it is doubtful that they even know, that we should be in a cooling period but our temperatures are spiking giving us record-breaking hot years nearly every year. Here is what the politicians do not tell us, either because of ignorance or deception.

Evidence from the last 5 million years of coring into the sediments of the oceans and the polar regions shows that, prior to 3 million years ago, even with the hundred thousand year variations, the average temperatures were higher than during the last 3 million years. They were higher still in the previous 60 million years. And now we are entering another cooling period but our temperatures are increasing faster than any time in the past. And CO_2 is leading the way.

The previously mentioned hundred-thousand-year cycle is due to the fact that the Earth's orbit around the sun is elliptical, not circular, and the orbit is elongated about every hundred thousand years. This makes the time that the Earth is near the sun shorter and the huge distances from the sun longer, resulting in longer cold periods.

But there are other cycles within this hundred-thousand-ear cycle. About every 41,000 years the landmass of the northern hemisphere tilts more toward the sun, then more away from the sun. Every 26,000 years there is a polar wobble that also exposes the landmass to or away from the sun. So we have a number of factors that change the climate that increases or decreases the amount of landmass that faces the sun or is farther from the sun. Then within these cycles the sun often gives off extra heat through sunspots or irradiance. This can cause more heat to reach the earth. So there is more to explain warming and cooling than just looking at a single temperature chart showing the last 60 million years.

GREENHOUSE GASES

We need some! Without a desirable amount of greenhouse gases our planet's temperature would be about 60 degrees Fahrenheit (33° Celsius) colder. Where would we go for a summer vacation? But we have fattened up our atmosphere with too many, and too much, of these good things. Just as on a vacation we may eat too much and fatten our bellies, our modern lifestyles have gorged our skies with gases to the point where we may become extinct. We should have listened to Aristotle, who advised us to take everything in moderation!

But our pursuit of the good life needs: bigger houses, more comfort producing gadgets, fossil fueled cars for every family member, more barbequed steaks, a television in every room, and—but you get the point! Then there are our distant vacations, international business travel, and all the other realities that make the good life possible.

SO WHY IS IT HAPPENING?

The sun heats the earth every day. Every night the heat escapes into our atmosphere. It should rise through the various levels of atmosphere and escape into space. Some gases reflect that heat back toward the Earth. This is good, or we would freeze every night. But if there is too much reflecting gas, the Earth will get warmer and warmer. That is the situation we find ourselves in today. We are living in a planetary greenhouse.

The name "greenhouse" comes from the greenhouses that are often used by farmers and horticulturists to speed the growth of plants by providing heat for more hours in a day. Below are photos of a home greenhouse and a commercial greenhouse. But, to get a similar effect, poorer farmers may use canvas, metal, or plastic roofing held up by wooden stakes to reduce the loss of the daytime heat at night.

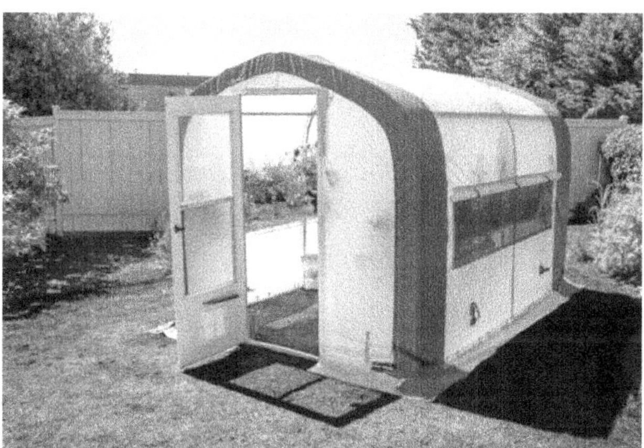

Home greenhouse for flowers, herbs, or vegetables.

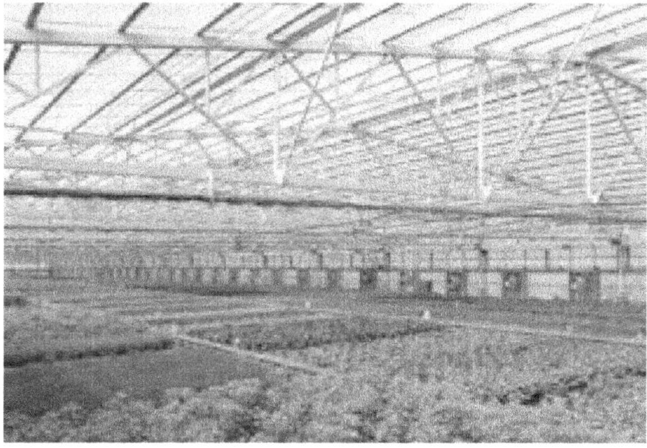

Large commercial greenhouse for vegetables

There are a number of gases in our atmosphere that reflect heat back to the earth. The most plentiful are: carbon dioxide (CO_2), water vapor (H_2O), methane (NH_3), nitrous oxide (N_2O), and ozone (O_3). On Earth, we have many uses for these compounds and molecules, among them are: carbon dioxide in carbonated drinks, ozone for cleaning our water, methane for powering some vehicles, and nitrous oxide as laughing gas.

A number of natural gases and solid particles, like soot, can escape the ground level and begin reflecting back the Earth's stored heat. This has resulted in a 45% increase in carbon dioxide in the last 270 years—since the Industrial Revolution began. In that period of time the carbon dioxide gas increased from 280 parts per million (ppm) of air, which had been the level for centuries, to 415 ppm in 2019. Most of this increase has been caused by burning fossil fuels—such as coal, oil, gasoline, and natural gas. To this has been added methane, from biomass decomposition and the flatulence of cows and other animals. Ozone (O_3) is a byproduct of the combustion of fuels from autos and industry. It is irritating to our mucous membranes at ground level and is a greenhouse gas at higher levels. There are also many man-made compounds including fluorine and the other elements that make the major greenhouse gases—carbon, oxygen, nitrogen, and hydrogen.

These greenhouse gases warm the air which makes it drier. Water vapor is evaporated from the oceans, lakes, and damp ground. This water vapor becomes the most potent greenhouse gas. It is short-lived, but easily replaced after it has been released as rain, snow, fog, or other moisture.

LOOKING AT OUR CLIMATE HISTORY

Ice-core analyses have extended the record back to 800,000 years with the same conclusion that the concentrations of these greenhouse gases were always lower before industrialization.

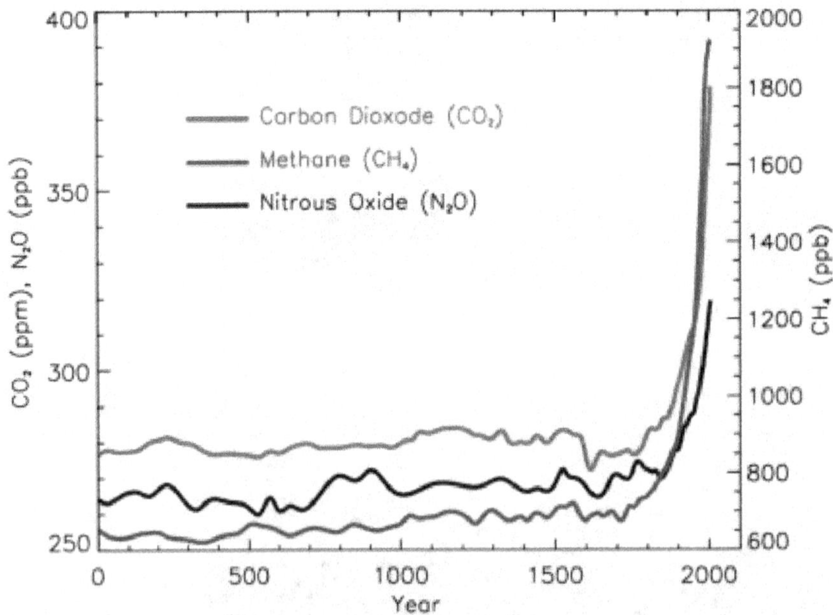

Carbon dioxide, CO_2 (the top line) is measured in parts per million in the air.

Nitrous oxide N_2O (middle line) and methane CH_4 (bottom line) are measured in parts per billion in the air. Values in the above figure for the past several decades are direct measurements of atmospheric composition. Earlier values are from ice-core analyses.

Should greenhouse gas emissions continue at their rate from 2019, global warming could cause Earth's surface temperature to exceed historical values as early as 2047, with potentially harmful effects on ecosystems, biodiversity and human livelihoods.

At current emission rates, temperatures could increase by 2°C, which the United Nations' IPCC designated as the upper limit to avoid "dangerous" levels, by 2036. Aside from water vapor, as mentioned, the four principal greenhouse gases are carbon dioxide (CO_2), methane (CH_4), nitrous oxide (N_2O) and the halocarbons or CFCs (gases containing fluorine, chlorine and bromine). These gases can remain in the atmosphere for different amounts of time, from months to millennia, and affect the climate on very different timescales. Some are measured in parts per million (ppm), some in parts per billion (ppb).

Gas	Concentration	Atmospheric Contribution to warming
Water vapor (incl. clouds)	10 to 50,000 ppm	36-72%
Carbon dioxide	400 ppm	9-26%
Methane	1.8 ppb	4-9%
Ozone	2-8 ppb	3-7%

The following chart shows some greenhouse gases, the amount of time they will remain in the atmosphere, and how much more harmful they are than carbon dioxide—which is given the value of 1.

	Lifetime in years in atmosphere	Multiple of CO_2 Damage 20 yrs	100 yrs
Carbon dioxide CO2	30-95	1	1
Methane CH4	10-12	84	28
Nitrous oxide N2O	121	264	265
Various fluorine compounds	1 to 50,000	450-16.000	150- 24,000

Many fluoride compounds are no longer used or being phased out because of the Montreal Accord, which found universal agreement that it was depleting the ozone layer. The other fluoride containing HCFC gases are to be phased out by 2030.

CARBON DIOXIDE (CO_2)

Carbon dioxide is the major long-lasting gas in the atmosphere. The most common estimate of its half-lifetime is 38 tears, but some estimate it to be as long as 200 years. The atmospheric CO_2 concentrations are now 415 ppm or more.

Although in itself not the most potent of the greenhouse gases, it is the gas that the IPCC (Intergovernmental Panel on Climate Change) has rated it as having the most warming effect therefore it's effects are the most damaging. Carbon dioxide is also the standard against which other gases are rated in the comparisons over a 100-year scale. (other gases are often measured on a scale of CO_2e (carbon dioxide equivalents.) The lifetime in the air of CO_2, the most significant man-made greenhouse gas, is probably the most difficult to determine, because there are several processes that remove carbon dioxide from the atmosphere. Between 65% and 80% of CO_2 released into the air dissolves into the ocean over a period of 20–200 years. The rest is removed by slower processes that take up to several hundreds of thousands of years.

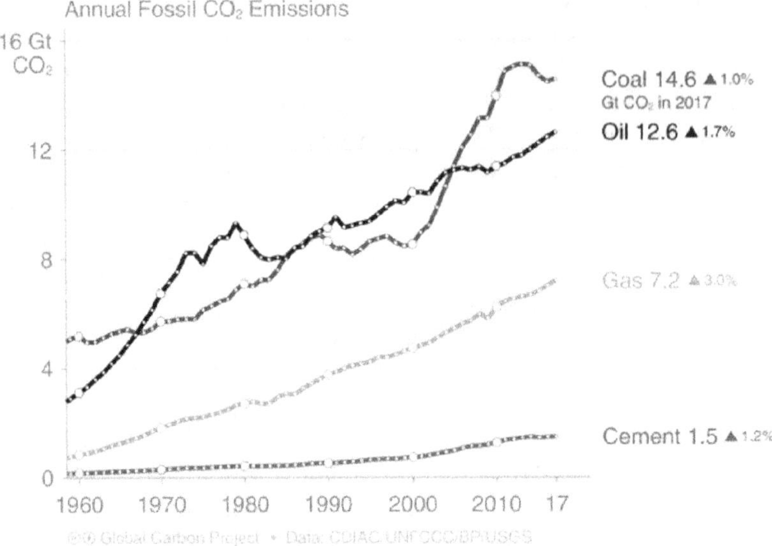

Once in the atmosphere, carbon dioxide can continue to affect the climate for many years.

In the economic realm, the estimates of economic costs of every ton of carbon dioxide that goes into the atmosphere or the oceans average $12 a ton, but the range of predictions is from $3 to $95 a ton. We know it's bad, but we don't know how bad.

Another area of economic estimates indicates that to stem the dangers of CO_2 it would take 1% of the gross domestic product to be invested in reducing carbon dioxide emissions, and if they are not sufficiently reduced a global recession of up to 20% of the world's gross domestic product will occur.

What about the carbon dioxide we exhale? The estimates are that humans exhale about 2 tons of carbon dioxide a year. That would be about 15 billion tons of CO_2 for the planet's population.

CARBON MONOXIDE (CO)

Of course, carbon monoxide is a byproduct of anything that is burned that contains carbon. That includes about every kind of combustion from candles and home fireplaces to cars and rockets. It's a deadly poison, which is why people often commit suicide by running the car in a locked garage and breathing in the fumes. Your red blood cells prefer carbon monoxide to oxygen, but your tissues need oxygen, and the oxygen in the carbon monoxide cannot be released into the blood. So if there is carbon monoxide in the air your blood cells latch on to it and your blood becomes oxygen starved. At 50 to 70 parts per million you can begin being poisoned and at two or three times that level you will probably be on your way to meeting your Maker.

In the atmosphere carbon monoxide will eventually combine with oxygen and become carbon dioxide. So whether you are burning wood in a fireplace or candles on your dinner table, you are contributing carbon monoxide and carbon dioxide to our atmosphere.

WATER VAPOR (H₂O)

Water vapor accounts for the largest percentage of the greenhouse effect, between 36% and 66% if the sky is clear and between 66% and 85% when clouds dot or cover the sky. Water vapor concentration is somewhat dependent on where one measures it in the world. Lakes, rivers and irrigated farmland will increase the potential that water vapor will be a warming factor. Air temperature is another variable. The warmer it is, the more water vapor the air can hold. At 32 degrees F (0 degrees C) the air can hold only 3% of water vapor.

You have probably heard the saying, "It's not the heat, it's the humidity."

Humans don't contribute much to the production of water vapor, but they do contribute directly to the warning that makes the air capable of absorbing the water.

The average residence time of a water molecule in the atmosphere is only about nine days, compared to years or centuries for other greenhouse gases such as CH_4 and CO_2.

METHANE (NH$_3$)

After carbon dioxide, the most significant greenhouse gas is methane. It accounts for 4 to 9% of the greenhouse effect. It has doubled in the atmosphere since the beginning of the industrial revolution.

Its major source is natural gas fields because natural gas is 97% methane. The oil and gas industries actually contribute 30% of the methane released into the atmosphere. When it is burned we produce more CO_2. About 10% of methane comes from biomass burning. Methane is also derived from things like rice paddies, bovine flatulence, bacteria in bogs, the thawing of the arctic tundra in Russia and Canada, the decomposition of garbage, and from fossil fuel production. Most of the world's rice, and all of the rice in the United States, is grown on flooded fields. When fields are flooded, anaerobic conditions develop and the organic matter in the soil decomposes, releasing methane, CH_4, into the atmosphere.

The Food and Agriculture Organization (FAO) of the United Nations reports that 14% of human related emissions come from livestock—about 7.1 billion tons (gigatons) of CO_2 equivalents come from livestock—41% from beef and 20% from milk cows. This does not include the emissions from their manure. Pigs contribute another 9% and chickens and eggs 8%. Then we would need to add in: the sheep and goats, dogs and cats, giraffes and zebras,--and don't forget the elephants! All are adding methane and CO_2.

A surprising study from Hawaii has found that plastic, like plastic bags—especially those made from polyethylene, like grocery bags—decompose and give off methane when in sunlight or seawater. It took about 152 days in seawater before the methane began to be released.

Although methane is about 200 times less abundant than carbon dioxide in the atmosphere, but molecule for molecule methane is 25 times more effective at trapping heat. It has a half-life of about ten to twelve years in the atmosphere. Since the beginning of the Industrial Revolution, methane has more than doubled in the troposphere. Additionally, its concentration has been increasing at about 1% per year.

Methane is mostly removed from the atmosphere by chemical reaction, which takes about 12 years. Thus, although methane is a potent greenhouse gas, its effect is relatively short-lived.

As the oceans warm we can expect methane, which has been trapped in the ice under the ocean's sediment, to be released. It is estimated that there are ten trillion tons which could be released. If they were all released at once we might expect another 5 degree increase in global temperature. More likely, is the release of methane from the peat bogs of the world where about 70 billion tons are stored.

OZONE (O$_3$)

Ozone is a relatively unstable molecule of three oxygen atoms. At ground level (tropospheric ozone) it is an air pollutant that is toxic to the respiratory system and to plants. At high altitudes, (upper tropospheric or stratosphere) 15 to 30 kilometers, it acts as a filter of harmful ultraviolet rays, reducing the number that reach the earth. But it also acts as a greenhouse gas trapping infrared rays reflected from the Earth. It accounts for 3 to 7% of the greenhouse effect.

NITROUS OXIDE (N_2O)

Then there's nitrous oxide, N_2O. You may have heard of the anesthetic called 'laughing gas', that's nitrous oxide. Nitrous oxide is naturally produced by oceans and rainforests. Man-made sources of nitrous oxide include nylon and nitric acid production, the use of fertilizers in agriculture, fossil fuel use, cars with catalytic converters, and the burning of organic matter—biomass burning. Agriculture is responsible for four and a half million tons per year. It is nearly 50% more prevalent now than before the industrial revolution.

Nitrous oxide is broken down in the atmosphere by chemical reactions that involve sunlight. Its concentrations have been increasing at about 0.3 percent per year for the last several decades. Yet, nitrous oxide has a lifetime of 150 years in the atmosphere, which contrasts sharply with the 10-year lifetime of methane. A single nitrous oxide molecule is the equivalent of 200 to 300 carbon dioxide molecules in terms of its greenhouse gas effect. Biomass burning accounts for about 2 to 3 percent of the total amount of troposphere nitrous oxide.

SULPHUR DIOXIDE (SO_2)

Acid rain is a major effect of excessive oxides of sulfur. Well over a third of China has been dampened by acid rain from the 25 million tons of sulfur dioxide emitted from their coal and oil burning factories. The Chinese output of sulfur dioxides is increasing at almost 10% per year. While the cheaper energy sources are good for business they harm the soil and vegetation. It's not a greenhouse gas, but it is certainly an air pollutant.

FLUORINATED GASES

Gases containing fluorine and carbon, sulfur, nitrogen or other elements, are man-made. They can last for thousands of years in the atmosphere, but at this time are a very small percentage of greenhouse gases.

CHAPTER 4
THE MAJOR POLLUTERS

How do various countries rank, per capita, in terms of CO_2 output?

The U.S.A. and China produce more CO_2 from fossil fuels and cement manufacturing than any other country—about 6 billion tons a year each. But China has more than three times as many people. Maybe we should look at it from a per capita output. When we do that we find that oil producing countries, like Qatar which heads the list with more than 40 metric tons per year, per-person. The smaller Arab Mideast states are also high, in the 20 plus metric ton range. But the US is right up there at over 16 metric tons per person. Canada is pretty high too, at about 15. Most of the European countries are in the 5 to 9 metric ton range. Mexico averages 4 tons per person which is below the world average of 5. Naturally the undeveloped countries range down to 0. Here are the 2014 World Bank ratings for some countries.

OIL PRODUCERS AND REFINERS
Bahrain 23.5, Brunei Darussalam 22.2, Oman 15.2, Qatar 43.9,
Saudi Arabia 19.4,
United Arab Emirates 22.9

HIGH POLLUTING COUNTRIES (Over 10 metric tons per person)
Australia 15.4, Canada 15.2, Estonia 14.8, South Korea 11.6, Russian Federation 11.9, Singapore 10.3, United States 16.5

MEDIUM PRODUCING COUNTRIES
Argentina 4.8, China 7.5, Czech Republic 9.2, Denmark 5.9, Finland 8.7, France 4.6, Germany 8.9, Iran 8.4, Iraq 4.9, Ireland 7.3, Israel 7.9, Italy 5.3, Japan 9.5, Mexico 4.0, Netherlands 9.9, New Zealand 7.7, Norway 9.3, South Africa 9.0, Spain 5.0, Sweden 4.5, Switzerland 4.3, United Kingdom 6.5

LOW PRODUCING COUNTRIES (Primarily Sub-Saharan and other undeveloped countries)
Afghanistan 0.3, Cambodia 0.4, Cameroon 0.3, Central African Republic 0.1, Ethiopia 0.1, India 1.7, North Korea 1.6, Rwanda 0.1, Somalia 0.0

What the list does not show is the contribution of each country from burning wood for cooking or heating, or the pollutants produced from forest fires or volcanoes.

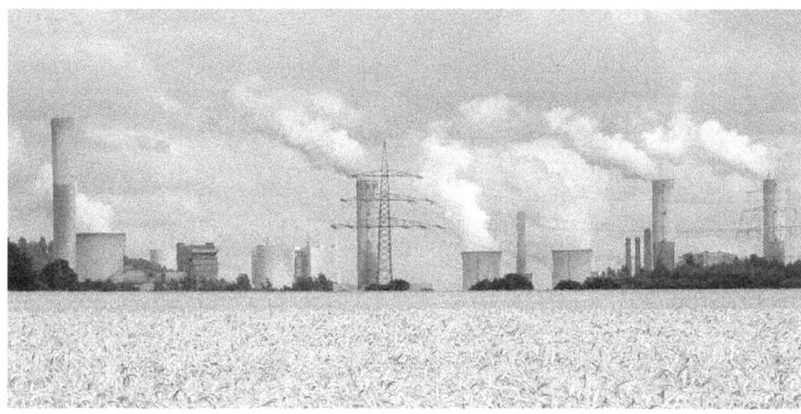

POLLUTANTS

Looking at the amount of CO_2 produced in generating one kilowatt hour of power from one kilogram (2.2 pounds) of fuel, we find that natural gas is the least polluting and burning wood is the most polluting.

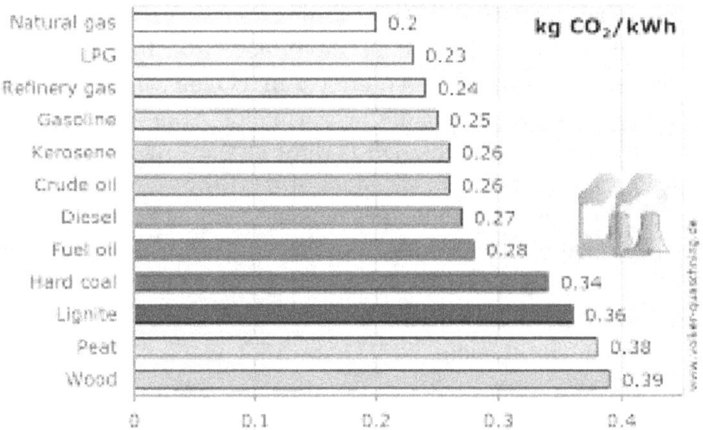

While writing this chapter in early October of 2019 I read an article in the Norwegian newspaper *Dagsavisen*. In an interview with the head of a wood consultancy, he was clear that burning wood was the least polluting fuel. Most homes in Norway have wood-burning fireplaces, In fact they are a "must" in every expensive home and every inexpensive cabin. Norwegians are leaders in fighting climate change. They allowed electric cars to be sold without the very high taxes on new cars. They allowed electric cars to park free when others had to pay for parking. They have companies selling solar power plants around the world. But how can burning wood cause pollution? "We have always done it." It's like Californians driving their cars 30 to 50 miles each way to work, with only the driver. "We've always done it!" But if we don't change our traditional habits, our children and grandchildren will be living in a far less hospitable world.

It goes without saying that the carbon that the trees capture for photosynthesis is reintroduced into the atmosphere. Then, as the charred remains decompose methane and oxides of nitrogen are released.

Approximate natural and human contributions to greenhouse gases in billions of tons per year.

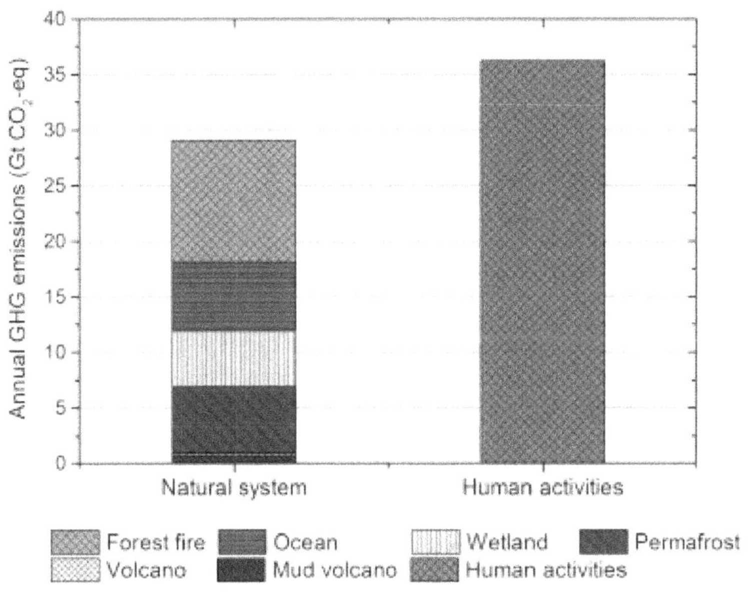

Greenhouse Warming Potential in grams CO₂-equivalent per passenger-kilometer

	URBAN	RURAL	HIGHWAY
Car (driving alone)	310	180	220
(with 1 passenger)	155	90	110
(with 3 passengers)	78	45	55
Motorcycles/scooters	260	190	330

AND A NEW CONCERN!

In an international study headed by the University of Southern California, and reported in Science Daily in February 2019, found that there are carbon and methane reservoirs on the ocean floor that can release the gases they harbor. These reservoirs are from undersea volcanoes and changes in the planetary crust. They are found in all oceans and they can be destabilized with increasing ocean temperature. One near Taiwan, is only a few degrees from destabilizing and releasing its gases.

These situations have been found in the Gulf of California, off the west coast of Canada, in the Aegean Sea, and other places around the Pacific rim. We don't know yet how many of these are vulnerable to destabilization because of ocean temperature rises. A newly found concern is that ocean heat has increased rapidly over the last 50 years. The oceans have retained 60% more heat than scientists had predicted.

History has shown that such destabilizations have occurred throughout history, the last was about 17,000 years ago. The undersea heating may have been responsible, in large part, for the ending of the last ice age. About 55 million years ago there was a huge jump in global temperatures, about 8°C higher than today.

Scientists have not yet mapped all the potential reservoirs and they do not know exactly how much warming will trigger the release of each of them. Additionally, the oceans are not equally warm in each geographic area nor at any particular depth.

CHAPTER 5
UNDERSTANDING OUR VALUES AND ETHICS—AND CONFLICTS IN OUR VALUES

The problems related to climate change, caused by global warming, should be obvious to everyone. Why aren't they? They are for most informed people, but even informed people may be more concerned with making money or being elected. So, let's look briefly at the kinds of values we may hold—and how important they are to us. The more important they are, the harder we will work to achieve them.

Our values come from three sources:

> Self-centered values,
> What we believe are God based values, and
> What we believe are values for the best society.

We can further understand them in terms of whether we are concerned with satisfying that value now or in the future.

SELF-CENTERED VALUES

> It is cold today so I buy a warm coat, that is self-centered with the present time as my major concern.

> If it is a warm July day and winter coats are on sale for half-price and I buy one, it is self-centered with the future in mind. I will use the coat when it is cold, and I will have more money in the future because I saved half of the winter price.

> Tomorrow I have a very important test in my ecology clas s, but there is an interesting party to which I have been invited. I choose to go to the party. This is self-centered with the present time as my major concern.

> I choose to study for the test. I want to learn more about ecology, and I might want to become an environmental engineer. So my actions were self-centered, with the future as my concern.

GOD-BASED VALUES

In the early verses of the Jewish Torah and the Christian Old Testament, this commandment appears, "Be fruitful and increase in number; fill the earth and subdue it. Rule over the fish in the sea and the birds in the sky and over every living creature that moves on the ground." Have we subdued the Earth yet?

The Qu'ran, of the Muslims, does not give such a command. Neither do Hindu scriptures.

SOCIETY-BASED VALUES

People living in Sweden are not immediately affected by climate change, but the major leader today in pushing for a change is a young Swede, Greta Thunberg. She is concerned for her future (self-centered value) and the future of the planet (a societal value).

Many people are concerned about climate change because it is causing the extinction of many species, destroying coral reefs, and negatively affecting our oceans and other bodies of water. These are purely societal values.

CONFLICTS IN VALUES

Obviously, in combatting climate change we are looking at what is good for society, however many, if not most, are concerned with themselves in their futures and for their children and grandchildren. So for most, it is a self-centered value with the future being of major concern.

Greta has been criticized for not knowing what she is talking about. She is, after all, a young girl being criticized by rich old men. Anyone with a basic knowledge of philosophy knows that this is a logical fallacy called *Argumentum ad hominem*— criticizing the person, rather than what is said.

If an idiot in a mental institution says that the Earth is round, or more correctly an "oblate spheroid' (a slightly flattened sphere) but the president of your country says that "the world is flat," it is the idiot, not the leader, who is correct! We see such fallacious arguments continually in politics, especially by the uninformed. (If you would like a more complete list of commonly used fallacious arguments, logical fallacies, see: "Revitalizing Demo cracy," a print book, or "Dumbing Down Demo cracy," an e-book—by the author.)

THE ASSUMPTIONS WE USE MAY VARY WITH THE VALUE WE ARE CONSIDERING

We all may hold values in each of these three different assumptions depending on the issue. Perhaps, when it is cold, I want to wear my mink coat-- even though many people believe that raising animals for their skins is immoral. I would be using a self-centered value. I may be a Catholic, so I am against abortion. This is obviously a God basis. At the same time, I may be working for the Green Party to reduce carbon dioxide pollution. This would be a society-based value. But it could also be a God-based value. Looking at a few verses from Genesis we can see some "God assumptions" implied:

➢ *1:26 "And God said, let us make man in our image, after our likeness: and let them have dominion over the fish of the sea, and over the fowl of the air, and over the cattle, and over all the earth, and over every creeping thing that creepeth upon the earth."*

➢ *1:28 "And God blessed them, and God said unto them, be fruitful, and multiply, and replenish the earth, and subdue it: and have dominion over the fish of the sea, and over the fowl of the air, and over every living thing that moveth upon the earth."*

If God gave dominion "over all the earth," and commanded us to "subdue" the earth, we could certainly make a case for a God basis here. But Genesis does not specifically mention climate change.

LET'S LOOK AT ANOTHER VALUE QUESTION IN AMERICAN SOCIETY

Let us look briefly at what may be America's major health prob lem-- the opioid addiction levels. What if we have a person we do not know who is a fentanyl addict, and has been for five years. He has been in treatment centers three times, but does not want to give up his habit because it feels so good. Should we just let him die on his next overdose?

His sister and mother want to protect him and hope he will give up his habit. Their desires are self-centered.

We have some people in the Salvation Army who have taken him into their shelters and fed him. Since all people are created in the image of God, all of us are equally valuable and the Salvation Army follows this ethical God-based idea.

On the other hand, there are people who believe that anyone who chooses to use addicting drugs is not worthy of the society. Why should our society spend police time, ambulance driver time, doctor and nurse time, on this derelict? We would be better off spending the money on schools and scholarships for people who have a good chance of helping society. After all, there is only so much money for society to use. So, where are the best places to put our tax dollars for the betterment of our society?

Is working to reduce climate change a goal for you? How much time and money are you willing to spend to make this value a reality? Are you willing to run for public office? Are you willing to spend time working for politicians who are honestly seeking to reverse climate change

CHAPTER 6
THE DENIERS

The evidence is so clear, and is affirmed by at least 97% of scientists who study the environment. Monitoring the air temperatures, the water temperature and the ocean acidity, the greenhouse gases in the atmosphere, the increase in forest fires and strong storms—all predictable—prove beyond a doubt that climate change is with us—and the evidence is, as scientists say, is highly probable. Probable like, the sun will come up in the east tomorrow morning-- or my mother-in-law will congratulate me tomorrow for being her daughter's best choice for a husband!

But what is the cause? There must be a cause! Is God angry with us? Is the magnetic North Pole shifting? Is it an increase in solar flares? It couldn't possibly be human caused! It couldn't possibly be that humans have created greenhouse gases that are heating this great big planet! As the evidence mounts to undeniable proportions, who could deny it? Imbeciles? Lunatics? Oil billionaires or the legislators they have bought?

It may surprise a few to realize that most of the scientist and legislative climate deniers are funded by fossil fuel interests. Can you believe that if we went totally green tomorrow the ExxonMobil, Chevron and Koch Industries would have no income. And we all know that there is nothing more important in life than money. Money gives us the best schools for our children, the best Scotch for our toddies, and the best politicians that money can buy.

The "Institute for Energy Research" is a scientifically sounding name. It does its best, without sound evidence, to downplay, not only climate change, but also solar and wind power. I wonder who finances this non-profit group? Oh my goodness! The early funding came from the oil billionaire Koch brothers. Exxon-Mobil was another funder that deducted its contributions to this anti-citizen pro-oil group. Some might wonder how its charitable non-profit status was approved!

It's about freedom. Freedom of belief—no matter how unlikely it is or how counter it is to scientific evidence. American have a Constitutional guarantee of free political speech that its Supreme Court has enlarged to give Americans the right

FREEDOM OF SPEECH

Freedom of speech, at the time of the Constitution's writing, was primarily a concern regarding freedom of political speech. However, the Supreme Court decisions have widened the scope of this freedom far beyond what the Founding Fathers had envisioned. Does freedom of speech have to be true or have evidence behind it or is it merely enough to use it to deflect the arguments on the issue? When President Trump said that Barack Obama had tapped his telephone lines during the election process, without presenting any evidence, is this what the writers of the Constitution meant to include in their "free speech" clause?

How important is free-speech for a democracy? And should the freedom have no limits? In 1969, in Brandenburg versus Ohio, the Court overturned several of its previous decisions, ruling that government cannot punish inflammatory speech unless that speech is "directed to inciting or producing imminent lawless action and is likely to incite or produce such action." This has been taken to mean that you can advocate harming a specific group tomorrow, but you can't advocate such violence for today, because "today" is "imminent."

In 2016, the New York Daily News reported that the Catholic Church had spent $2.1 million in lobbying to block legislation that would make it easier for victims of child abuse by priests to sue the church. About the same time, Catholic churches in Pennsylvania were advising their parishioners of the evil legislators who had voted for bills that would protect abused children. These lobbying expenses seem to be illegal according to the Tax Code, but who wants to sue God?

So what about oil and coal companies paying legislators and plying their anti-planet, anti-humanity propaganda? Should utter falsehoods and self-serving lies or hate speech be allowed? Most European countries have limitations on saying anything you want—like profanity or extreme political views, like Nazism, racism and other forms of hate speech.

FREEDOM OF THE PRESS

Freedom of the press similarly was concerned with political freedom, and we might say, the freedom to criticize the government and its policies. In early 2017 Trump blocked some media outlets from a White House press briefing. They included: the New York Times, the LA Times, and CNN. Was this a violation of this amendment?

These last two ideas, of freedom of speech and freedom of the press, may have been overly stretched in the American presidential campaign of 2016. Fake news, fake history, opinions portrayed as news, the criticism of the legitimate press, as well as the lies and faulty logic that were exhibited certainly took the election far adrift of meaningful intellectual and logical discussions. How much should propaganda be protected in a democratic election?

In April of 2018, the Reporters Without Borders released their latest World Press Freedom Index. The United States fell two places to 45th in the world. Not quite what Jefferson and Madison had envisioned. Who was first? Yes, it was Norway leading the world. It was followed by: Sweden, the Netherlands, Finland, and Switzerland. Is it merely an accident that the happiest countries in the world, according to the United Nations' Happiness Index, are also: the least corrupt, have the greatest press freedom, have the most democratic governments, have students that achieve higher, have inexpensive or free universities, and have less crime? But that isn't really a concern for us Americans. Give us low taxes and let our children pay off the debts we have incurred! Forget promoting the general welfare with a free press, I only want to hear what I want to hear. How else can we out-Fox our opposition?

Why should you worry? We're all going to die eventually, as David Koch did recently.

The Kochs, David and Charles, have given over $1.2 billion to libertarian causes. And we would have to agree with them and the Libertarian Party. Why should we have taxes, especially income taxes. And, you would probably agree with them that we should eliminate: the I.R.S., the F.B.I., the C.I.A., the Environmental Protection Agency, the Food and Drug Administration, and the S.E.C. And who needs public education? Medicare and Social Security cost the billionaires way too much money in taxes. And who needs child labor laws or minimum wages?

When the brothers have $120 billion, after taking out their lunch money, there is enough left over to convince or bribe people to see their position—that it is good to let them keep their fortunes. They therefore found and/or fund a number of organizations geared to allowing them to keep and increase their fortunes. What could be more American than that? Here are some of their major propaganda generating think tanks and institutes: <u>Cato Institute</u> which Charles cofounded in 1977, <u>Americans for Prosperity</u>, founded by David Koch himself and which spent $40 million on the 2010 Congressional elections. It was certainly essential to slow or stop Obamacare. Then there are: the

American Enterprise Institute, the <u>George C Marshall Institute</u>, the <u>Reason Foundation,</u> the <u>Heritage Foundation</u>, and the <u>Manhattan Institute</u>.

Of course, the Kochs, other oil billionaires, and the individuals or companies with fortunes, are perfectly entitled to have their desires. Climate change will not affect them as much as it does us! They can always stay ahead of the problem. I understand that they are now buying beachfront property in Greenland!

CONFRONTING YOUR DENYING FRIENDS

How many temperature measuring stations do they have on land and in the oceans?

Those of us who believe in warming, base our evidence on over 1000 reporting stations on land and sea that have been recording temperatures for 50 to 100 or more years.

There are today 31,000 weather stations in the world.

The Climatic Research Unit of East Anglia University in the UK has charted the major reporting stations used by the IPCC.

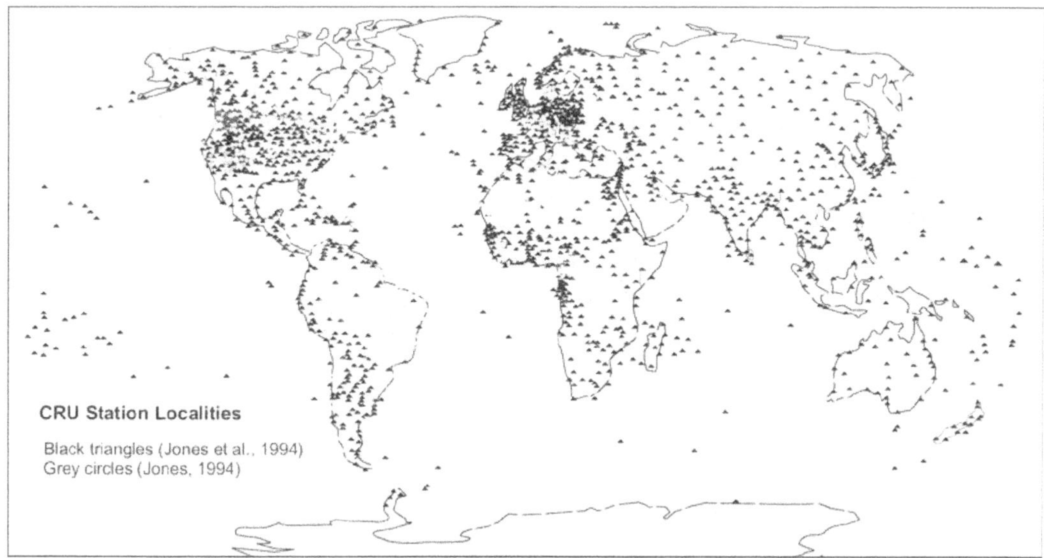

Temperatures from many years ago are only estimates deduced from ice cores and tree rings. With the invention of a thermometer with a scale was accomplished by Daniel Fahrenheit in 1714. Anders Celsius invented his 100 degree scale in 1742. These allowed for accurate temperature measuring.

In 1880, about 140 years ago, America began a more comprehensive recording of temperatures in the U.S. There had already been records kept. England also had been keeping records of land and sea temperatures throughout their Commonwealth.

A bit over ten years ago it was publicized that some thermometers were located in areas that would register a higher than actual temperature for the location. Being placed by an air conditioning outlet that was exhausting the warm air from a building, or placing it near a black asphalt parking area that radiates daytime absorbed temperatures into the nighttime air—raising the average temperature for the location. These poorly placed thermometers have been relocated to register true temperatures. The deniers made the few poorly-placed thermometers a very big deal. They really didn't inflate the mean temperatures, but now after their removal, the 1,000+ thermometers still show the steep increase of yearly temperatures.

CO2 Levels and Global Warming

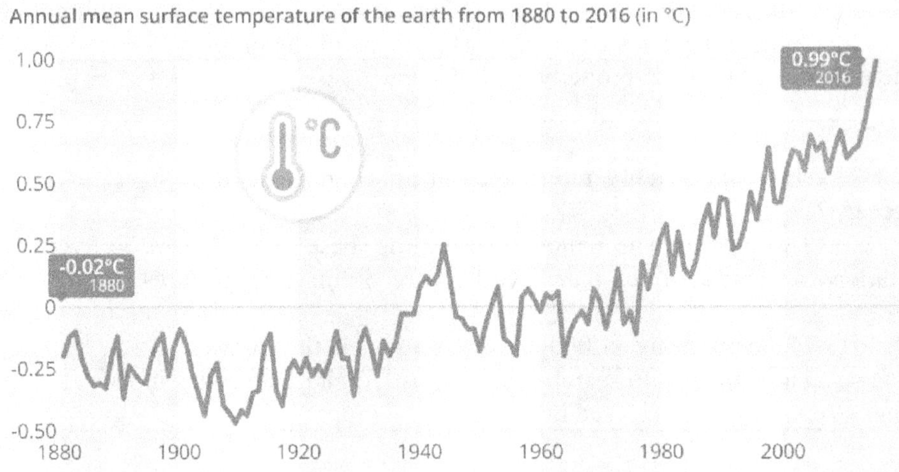

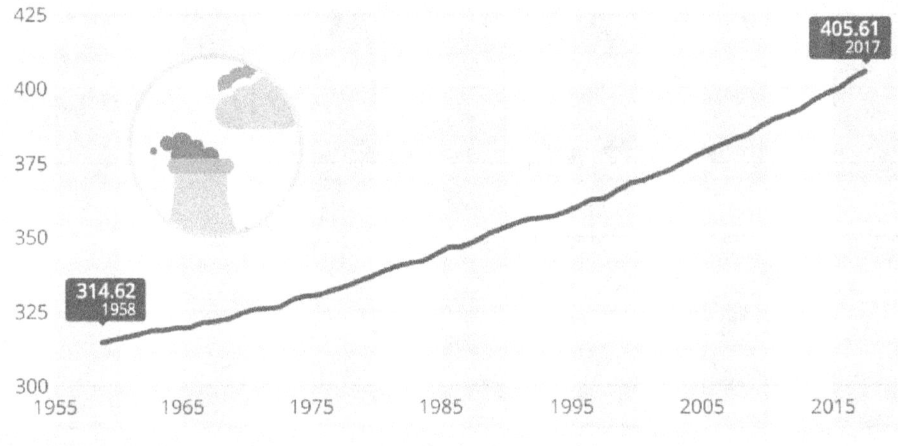

WHAT IS THE HISTORY OF THE REALITY?

In 1824, French scientist Joseph Fourier found that the planet was warmer than it should be based on its distance from the sun. This was called the "greenhouse effect." He hypothesized that the atmosphere must be retaining some of the sun's heat. In 1896, Swedish scientist Svante Arrhenius realized that CO_2 from coal burning was increasing considerably and was warming the world. So, if in 1900 we would have projected the warming, we might have done something then. But it was seen, by those few who noticed it, that it would be an advantage for crop production.

In 1938, British scientist Guy Callendar found that in the previous 45 years, the Earth had warmed Celsius (nearly one degree F). He noted that in that time, carbon dioxide had increased 10% during that period. He assumed that it was the product of the Industrial Revolution. So what! No politician would bring up scare mongering—even if he knew it existed.

In 1957, American scientist Roger Revelle found that the ocean was becoming more acidic due to its absorption of carbon dioxide. The population was exploding and each person was using more carbon dioxide producing energy. Then a colleague at Scripps, Charles Keeling, began monitoring CO_2 in the atmosphere. He found that the gas had increased from 280 parts per million to 315. It is more than 410 ppm today.

By the 1960s scientific voices were raising concerns of warming. Research into the area multiplied. In the 70s still more scientific voices were raised with concern. But who could believe such scare tactics. We certainly don't want to tamper with our economy or raise our taxes!

As the research deepened, more greenhouse gases were discovered.

People started to become aware when Al Gore started his speaking tours and released his Academy Award winning film, "Inconvenient Truth."

But money is more important than facts for legislators. And money does buy politicians. This reality is not lost on the energy companies.

ENERGY LOBBYIST CONTRIBUTIONS 2019

Contributor	Amount
Koch Industries	$1,943,933
Marathon Petroleum	$1,939,982
Chevron Corp	$1,459,904
Midland Energy	$1,322,678
Energy Transfer Partners	$1,265,269
Energy Transfer Equity	$1,100,000
Walter Oil & Gas	$1,037,900
National Rural Electric Cooperative Assn	$847,001
Parman Capital Group	$820,669
Nextera Energy	$738,686
Exelon Corp	$710,268
Otis Eastern	$704,297
Exxon Mobil	$554,463
Red Apple Group	$538,596
Occidental Petroleum	$502,493
Petroplex Energy	$500,000
Valero Services	$500,000
Hilcorp Energy	$497,684
Berexco Inc	$496,000
Hunt Companies	$413,640

Contributions to: Democrats

Republicans

Liberal Groups

Conservative Groups

Nonpartisan

The Kochs gave all their money to Republicans, as did several other energy companies. 13 gave 90 to 100% to Republicans. None gave more to the Democrats. Does this tell you anything about how our "democratic" system works?

In case you are interested, energy lobbyists are not the most generous in Washington. You might wonder why business, real estate, and social media get the tax breaks they do. Without their taxes the government has less money to spend on greenhouse gas reduction and research on renewable energy. Climate change spending, as you can see, is not a "one issue" factor.

Highest lobbying spenders.

US Chamber of Commerce	$94,800,000
National Assn of Realtors	$72,808,648
Open Society Policy Center	$31,520,000
Pharmaceutical Research & Manufacturers of America	$27,989,250
American Hospital Assn	$23,937,842
Blue Cross/Blue Shield	$23,884,221
Business Roundtable	$23,160,000
Alphabet Inc	$21,770,000
American Medical Assn	$20,427,000
AT&T Inc	$18,529,000
Boeing Co	$15,120,000
Comcast Corp	$15,072,000
Amazon.com	$14,400,000
Northrop Grumman	$14,390,000
National Assn of Broadcasters	$14,170,000
NCTA The Internet & Television Assn	$13,240,000
Lockheed Martin	$13,205,502
Facebook Inc	$12,620,000
Bayer AG	$12,310,000
Southern Co	$12,300,000

And you wondered why we don't have less expensive and better health care

SENATORS AND REPRESENTATIVESWHO TAKE LOBBYIST MONEY?

Recipient	From Lobbyists	From Lobbyists and Family Members
Kevin McCarthy (R-Calif)	$364,055	$364,055
Mitch McConnell (R-Ky)	$235,868	$262,068
Cory Gardner (R-Colo)	$220,475	$234,825
Gary Peters (D-Mich)	$214,590	$229,690

Recipient	From Lobbyists	From Lobbyists and Family Members
Steve Scalise (R-La)	$209,749	$210,249
Thom Tillis (R-NC)	$206,099	$219,449
John Cornyn (R-Texas)	$197,606	$201,356
Jeanne Shaheen (D-NH)	$192,055	$198,155
Doug Jones (D-Ala)	$181,161	$189,561
Richard E Neal (D-Mass)	$173,310	$179,310
Mark Warner (D-Va)	$164,998	$174,638
Ed Markey (D-Mass)	$148,997	$168,497
Susan Collins (R-Maine)	$105,276	$112,486
Lindsey Graham (R-SC)	$101,775	$101,975
Dan Sullivan (R-Alaska)	$97,458	$100,083
Greg Walden (R-Ore)	$95,286	$96,786
Steven Daines (R-Mont)	$90,733	$93,233
David Perdue (R-Ga)	$85,295	$85,545
Tina Smith (D-Minn)	$85,050	$87,850
Hakeem Jeffries (D-NY)	$84,971	$87,671
Dick Durbin (D-Ill)	$81,770	$82,770
Nancy Pelosi (D-Calif)	$81,265	$91,665
Ben Ray Lujan (D-NM)	$81,100	$81,100
Bradley Byrne (R-Ala)	$79,000	$79,000
Chris Coons (D-Del)	$78,500	$80,950
Steny H Hoyer (D-Md)	$77,600	$78,600
Frank Pallone Jr. (D-NJ)	$77,250	$77,250
Martha McSally (R-Ariz)	$73,833	$79,433
Amanda Makki (R-Fla)	$73,108	$75,608
Darin LaHood (R-Ill)	$71,450	$71,450
James M Inhofe (R-Okla)	$70,433	$73,983
George Holding (R-NC)	$68,621	$68,621
Jack Reed (D-RI)	$66,263	$67,263
Kevin Brady (R-Texas)	$61,502	$64,302

Recipient	From Lobbyists	From Lobbyists and Family Members
Steve Bullock (D)	$61,391	$63,416
Drew Ferguson (R-Ga)	$61,300	$61,300
Patrick McHenry (R-NC)	$60,950	$60,950
Ken Calvert (R-Calif)	$60,938	$60,938
Xochitl Torres Small (D-NM)	$60,079	$60,079
Pat Toomey (R-Pa)	$58,482	$59,982
Joni Ernst (R-Iowa)	$58,449	$58,949
Vernon Buchanan (R-Fla)	$57,121	$57,121
Devin Nunes (R-Calif)	$56,821	$56,821
Liz Cheney (R-Wyo)	$56,800	$56,800

If you wonder why 91 of the Fortune 500 American companies paid no income tax last year you can understand why—the legislators are bought and paid for. Amazon, IBM, DowDuPont, Levi Strauss, Whirlpool, US Steel, FedEx, Netflix, Chevron, and Delta Airlines If you wonder are examples. But don't worry, Donald Trump just borrowed the money to run the government--$2,700,000,000 ,0 0 0—$2.7 trillion. So every American family owes about $170,000 on that debt and the interest on it-- $480 billion, which is about 10% of the federal budget. But don't tax us now, borrow and let our children be taxed in the years ahead when we are retired! Oh! Oh! Maybe we can't retire because the government has borrowed most of the money from the government retirement funds, like Social Security.

Doesn't it make you feel all warm and cuddly, knowing that the richest of us can buy off our legislators, saddle us and our progeny with huge debts while helping to insure our climate changing demise. But never fear—they will survive, sunbathing in Vladivostok and surfing in Iceland. But how long will they keep denying climate change? Maybe when their fossil fuel using customers have all died from famines, fires, hurricanes and water wars!

But we must remember that the non-caring objective of modern self-centered capitalism is to make as much money as you can, and let the devil take this hindmost! Truth is not a concern, sitting on a mound of gold is the reason for our existence.

These companies have the money to control many legislators—BUT, we have the voting power to elect effective representatives.

CHAPTER 7
FINDING SOLUTIONS

It goes without saying that increasing the economic output of a nation and a higher standard of living for more people are the causes of much of climate change. Cheap coal is developing energy for countries like India and China. And the oil producing countries meet the desires of the richer countries for more of the comforts of life, for the people with money, around the world. But why live if we can't have a car for every member of our family? Why live if we can't have heating and air conditioning, big steaks and Big Macs, five bedroom homes and luxury travel?

Scientists will find a way to eliminate greenhouse gases and the nearly 8 billion people who produce them. And if they don't find solutions fast enough, Mother Nature will handle it with floods, famines, hurricanes, forest fires, wars, pestilences, terrorism, or other troubles that she and Pandora have in their bag of tricks.

The higher the income, the more CO_2 is produced because of the amenities of money: driving, air conditioning, consuming food requiring more energy to produce, living in bigger houses (energy cost of building materials), air travel, etc. A 2017 study from the London School of Economics reported that rich households in the United States in 2009, on average, created 12 metric tons of carbon dioxide per year just from driving their cars and a total of 59 tons of CO_2 for the entire household. A poor U.S. household creates about 18 metric tons in a whole year, including 3.6 metric tons from driving. So, the rich household is three times as much of a polluter than the poor family. During the period of the study, 1996 to 2009, the average household emissions dropped 10%, to 40 metric tons annually. This was attributed to more fuel-efficient cars and cleaner power generation.

THE EFFECTIVENESS OF ALTERNATE ENERGY SOURCES

Energy obviously costs money. There are the costs to build: the mines, the nuclear reactors, the wind turbines, the solar panels, etc. Then there are the salaries of: the miners, the inspectors, the assemblers, the researchers, and the maintenance personnel. Taking all of these into consideration in determining the cost of a kilowatt or megawatt hour, is called the "levelized cost of energy" (LCOE). Below is a graph showing the rapidly reducing cost of wind energy.

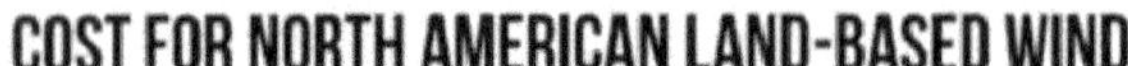

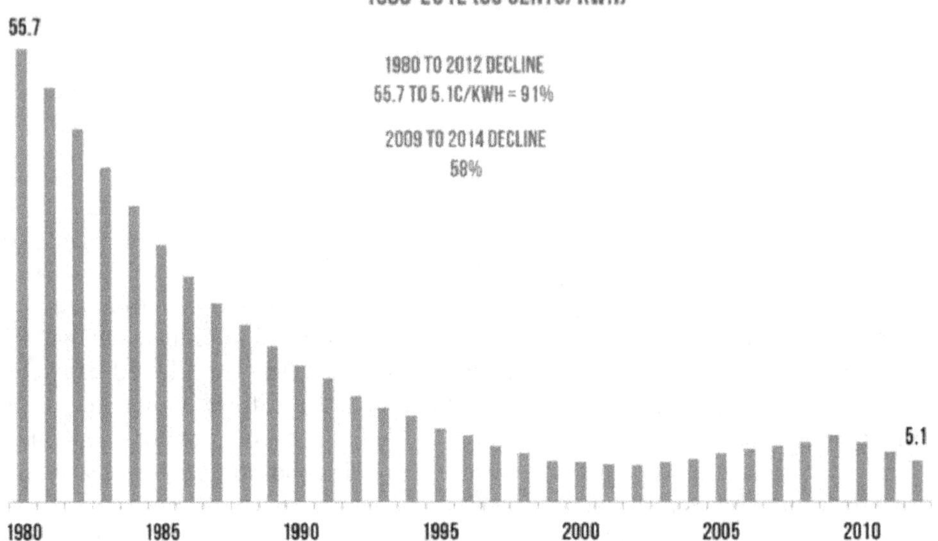

Bloomberg New Energy Finance (2019) estimated that photovoltaic solar power had decreased in price 81% in ten years, to $57 per megawatt hour (MWh). During the same period, land based turbines had fallen 46% to $50 per MWh and ocean based turbines had dropped 44% to $89 per MWh.

It is easy to see why photovoltaic energy is rapidly reducing in price. This Bloomberg chart shows the unbelievable decrease in the cost of the solar cells.

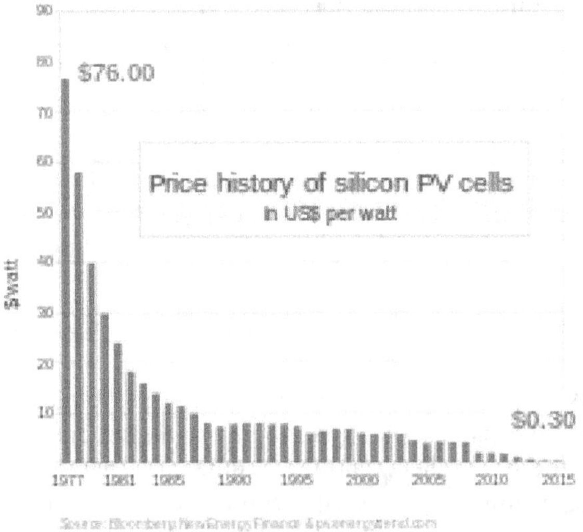

In spite of the probable cost of battery storage for the energy from the intermittent energy sources of the wind and the sunlight, batteries are being developed to handle them. The generated electricity may be stored many ways. For example, The electricity can power a pump to bring water uphill. Then when power is needed the water can flow downhill and turn a turbine to create electricity. Batteries use chemicals to store potential energy. They generally work with a DC output, but it can be charged with AV current. (Thomas Edison wanted to use only direct current for all uses but Nicola Tesla and George Westinghouse won the major battle for universal electricity, using alternating current.)

In October of 2018 the president of the World Bank said, "We are required by our by-laws to go with the lowest cost option, and renewables have now come below the cost of [fossil fuels]."

With these factors in mind, we know that renewable sources for energy cost less than fossil fuel produced energy. Then when we factor in the additional costs of fossil fuels, like the:

> ➤ Damage done to agriculture from acid rain,
> ➤ Damage to cities, farmland, and low lying islands from the rising oceans,
> ➤ Increasingly non-livable heat of lands closer to the equator,
> ➤ Increased storms (rain, snow, and wind) caused by the increased greenhouse gases,
> ➤ Increased forest fire danger

We have trillions of dollars in past and future expenses. Demonstrations for renewable energy should be easily mounted and easily accepted by the governments—BUT:

> ➤ Fossil fuel billionaires and industries have more money to influence legislators than do student and citizen protesters,
> ➤ The multi-million dollar lobbyist contributions to political parties and candidates is a formidable foe—It is a matter of educating citizens to do the things that will benefit them, rather than the things that will benefit non-caring billionaires and politicians.
> ➤ We must be prepared for the illogical warfare of propaganda, lies and other fake news, and the charges that we are: anti-capitalistic, anti-democratic, socialistic or other epithets that are born of the financially fueled fossil fuel spokespeople's propaganda.
> ➤ We must therefore:
>> • Find intelligent, well-educated, globally concerned people to run for legislative and executive positions around the world,
>> • Be knowledgeable about the facts,
>> • Organize the masses of concerned citizens to educate the voters in door-to-door encounters,
>> • If you believe that this book will aid in people's education, it will always be available free, as an e-book, through channels that accept free books, such as: Apple, Google, Smashwords, Kobo—and through the publisher totalhealthpublications.com.
>> • Print copies are available through all distributers.

As it stands now, controlling climate change will require inconveniences that many do not like—and will not accept! But which is the greater inconvenience, taking public transportation or dying??

The solutions range from individual to societal changes, which are achievable, and to population reduction, which is probably not achievable.

- ➢ INDIVIDUAL CHANGES—Can be done immediately
- ➢ SOCIETAL CHANGES—Can be done in a few years—but not fast enough to save all of us
- ➢ POPULATION REDUCTION—Too much resistance to this—Solution is likely to be total or extensive annihilation.

The first two can be started now.

INDIVIDUAL ACTIONS YOU CAN DO

Let first look at personal changes we can make immediately. Then we will look at international and national efforts and how near term economic issues inhibit the life or death issues of climate change. After we have done this we will look at the realities of the elephant in the room—overpopulation--and suggest some long-term solutions. However, traditions, both religious and societal, cannot be made fast enough to prevent the billions of deaths that could have been prevented if we had acted forcefully and decisively when we were first made aware of global warming.

People don't realize the environmental costs of the energy they use. For example, to burn a 100 watt bulb for a year, day and night, would use 714 pounds of coal or 143 pounds of natural gas or 32 hours of solar power from a 100 square meters of solar panels.

If every American would replace just one 100 watt light bulb with an energy saving bulb it would save enough energy to light 3 million homes for a year and would save nearly $700 million in annual energy bills. It would also reduce the greenhouse gas output by 4,500,000 tons about the equivalent of 800,000 cars. But we Americans are too self-centered, I'm afraid.

YOU CAN:

- ➢ Buy products with minimal packaging.
- ➢ Recycle paper, glass and other recyclables.
- ➢ Wash clothes in cold or warm water—saving up to 500 pounds of carbon dioxide.
- ➢ Turn off lights and appliances, TV, etc. when not in use.
- ➢ Conserve water by: taking shorter showers, using less water to water lawns, wash cars, etc.
- ➢ Start a plant-based diet with less meat. Reducing beef and dairy products and lamb, in favor of fish and chicken, not only helps the environment—it also gives you a much higher quality of protein. (Proteins are rated according to the amount of the various amino acids available. Egg whites are 96% perfect. Skim milk is 92, fish in the high 80s, chicken in the mid-80s, then organ meats, then steak in the high 70s. Beans come below that. But by combining some vegetables, such as wheat and peanuts (ie, peanut butter sandwich on whole wheat bread), or rice and beans (a Mexican tradition) high levels of protein can be achieved.
- ➢ Avoid palm oil and generic vegetable oils. Palm oil not only is high in the unhealthy saturated fats, but it is generally grown in areas of Malaysia and Indonesia where carbon sink forests have been burned down to clear the area for palm orchards where the oil is produced.
- ➢ Reduce food waste. Wasted food used water and fertilizer to produce. Estimates are that the power to produce that wasted food resulted in more than 50 gigatons (50 million tons) of carbon dioxide.
- ➢ Buy tax credits for your own emissions.
- ➢ Plant trees and other vegetation.

➢ You can also donate to charities that plant trees. For example, Eden Reforestation hires local residents to plant trees in Madagascar and Africa for $0.10 a tree. It also gives the very poor people an income, rehabilitates their habitat, and saves species from mass extinction. They report that they have planted 242 million trees and created two and a half million days of work,

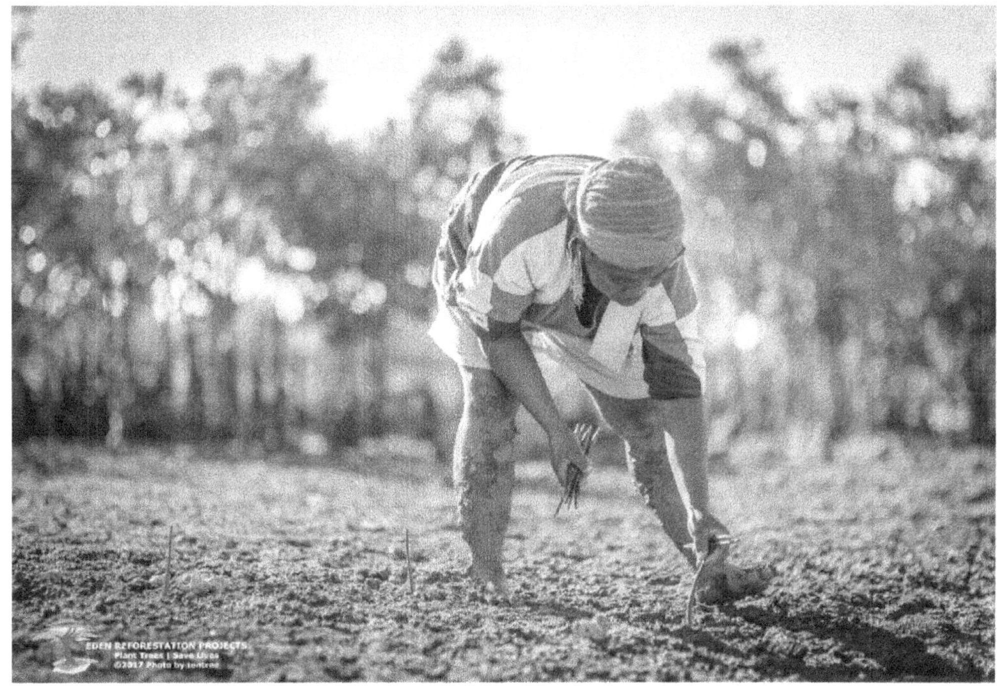

100 mangrove trees can absorb 2.18 metric tons of CO_2 annually. The average American would need to plant 734 mangrove trees to offset one year's worth of CO_2. At $0.10 a tree, that would cost $73.

Depending on the size of the tree, a proportional amount of carbon dioxide will be absorbed. Also, trees don't seem to have their growth enhanced if there is more CO_2 in the air, according to a major Swiss study.

YOUR HOME
➢ Check to see if solar water heaters would be helpful in your area.
➢ Check to see if photovoltaic panels are appropriate for your area.
➢ If your power company offers an energy audit—take them up on it.
➢ Turn your heating thermostat so that the heater comes on at a lower temperature. (Just find a sweater!) Turn it down at night. A $2°$ change saves about a ton of carbon dioxide per year.
➢ Turn your air conditioning thermostat so that it comes on at a higher temperature.
➢ Use solar or wind power for your home. Depending on the cost of the panels and installation and the cost of electricity from the local utility—the 20 year savings should be between $10,000 and $40,000.
➢ Insulate the walls.
➢ Caulk the exterior doors, windows, and any spaces that may let in outside air.
➢ Use double or triple paned windows.

➢ Install a programmable thermostat.
➢ Use florescent or LED light bulbs. Each will save energy and save you about $30 during its lifetime.
➢ When buying appliances, buy the energy efficient ones.
➢ Set your water heater thermostat at 120°.
➢ Wrap insulation around older water heaters.
➢ Buy low flow shower heads and water conserving toilets.

TRANPORTATION (Every gallon of gasoline not used saves 20 pounds of CO_2, so cut gasoline usage.
➢ Cycle when you can—without music in your ears.
➢ Use public transportation.
➢ Carpool
➢ Keep tires inflated properly
➢ Change the carburetor air filter often.
➢ Walk.

WORKING IN GROUPS TO INFLUENCE BUSINESS AND GOVERNMENT

Demonstrations do help to force business and governmental leaders to take a look at the problem. The weekly Hong Kong demonstrations, protesting the possible extradition of Hong Kong citizens to China, did not gain the withdrawal of the bill until the demonstrations had continued every weekend for three months. They became violent occasionally. The violence was probably a political mistake.

Continued demonstrations around the world this year have had some effect, especially in Lebanon where they were protesting a 20 cent tax on WhatsAp calls. They were also protesting corruption. (If the world's citizens wanted to protest corruption, we would have more that 7 billion protesters on the streets every day!)

Youth street protests, like those in the Arab Spring, and more recently in Lebanon, Chile, Venezuela and Hong Kong, sometimes get results. With all the Arab Spring protests, it seems that only those in Tunisia were really fruitful. In Palermo, Sicily, one judge who ruled against the mafia was murdered, another has been threatened with death. Huge groups of citizens held mass demonstrations against the mafia, and some volunteered as citizen bodyguards for the threatened judge.

So to be effective today, the protests need to be organized, continual, peaceful, and have leaders who really understand the problems and have realistic solutions. Legislators and presidents in democratic countries want to be re-elected—and most of them want more money in their pockets. Demonstrations and door-to-door voter re-education should be a goal. But then, how will you take on the energy companies and their millionaire and billionaire owners who are likely to oppose you with data-mining, social media, propaganda, and media ads?

Adult revolutionary actions, like the American and French revolutions, had major results. But today's governments have far more firepower than any revolutionary forces can muster. So the "free India" marches of Gandhi and the "free the Blacks" marches of Martin Luther King accomplished, peacefully, the objectives of the people.

In our modern democratic republics, it is possible to re-educate or replace representatives. But since they are often in the pockets of oil producers or energy-using industrialists, powerful grassroots green-advocates must use their time, and personal contact with voters, to counteract the data-mining and advertising of the opposition—those putting THEIR PROFITS over OUR LIVES.

OUR GOVERNMENTS

So what might we ask for?

Tax the rich-- but don't tax me! Is that really fair? In 2018-19 the President of France enacted a tax on vehicle fuel to tax the polluters. A grassroots "Yellow Vest" movement started in many cities. 500,000 people are said to have been involved. The tac was withdrawn. As President Macron said, "The end of the month bills won over the end of the world reality."

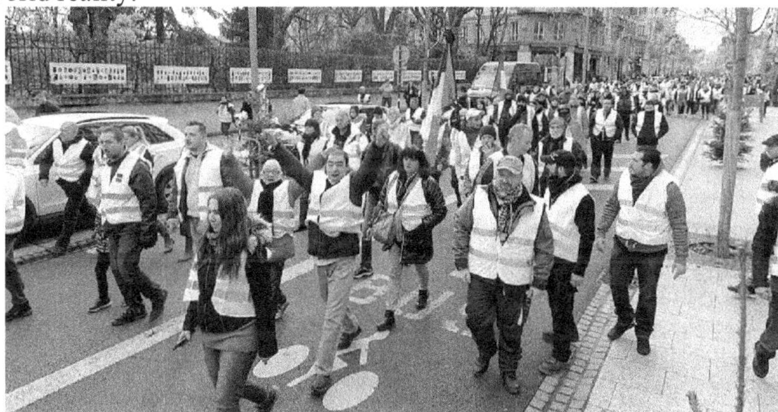

Impose very high carbon taxes on products manufactured with energy from fossil fuels, such as in India and China. Since the taxes will actually be paid by the consumer because the taxes or tariffs are merely added to the price of the goods, are you willing to pay those taxes?

Require individuals to buy tax credits for their own emissions---gasoline and utility taxes could handle this.

100% tax on inheritance for rich and poor, with free education for all in state universities. It is certainly possible that some poor kids might find some solutions for global warming—they might be more motivated to find some answers since they didn't have air conditioning in their homes—or tents!

Higher taxes to pay for research into alternate energy and water sources,

All countries, except the U.S., must make changes, because we don't want to burden the U.S. economy with carbon taxes, or the cost of using cleaner energy—and we can't use taxpayer money to pay for planting trees, in fact we should open more national forests for logging! Cutting down large carbon-absorbing trees must be good for the environment—or for some millionaires! At the same time, the developed world still gives China and India leeway in allowing their economic needs to use coal fired energy. Certainly, the economic development of most countries is more important than the lives of the people in all countries—and their progeny!

BUSINESS

Businesses sometimes take the responsible path on becoming carbon neutral, but the selfishness of both sole proprietors and stockholders generally require government regulation.

The United Nations program "Climate Neutral Now" allows businesses and individuals to offset their emissions by purchasing credits. These credits fund green initiatives, such as wind energy or solar power plants in developing countries.

GOVERNMENT REGULATION

Pressure for governmental action may be the major potential outcome of the Extinction Rebellion demonstrations. The ideal, of course, would be to have legislators and executives who understand the risks of climate change, who are not beholden to the energy industries, and who have no financial interests, such as stocks, in energy companies.

Some states are making exemplary progress. A bill signed by Nevada Gov. Steve Sisolak last year required utilities to get half of their electricity from renewable sources by 2030, and set a goal of 100% zero-carbon electricity by 2050. NV Energy, which is owned by Buffett's Berkshire Hathaway Energy and is the state's largest power provider, estimated that 24% of its electricity came from renewables in 2018. Several large solar farms are already operating near Las Vegas, with more on the way. California also has a number of large solar farms.

But we need to pressure corporations to disclose and act on their climate-related risks. 100 companies are responsible for more than 70% of greenhouse gas emissions. The worst are: ExxonMobil, Shell, BP, and Chevron. The necessary solutions require that the profits of companies and countries be required to bow to the necessity of self-preservation. While Genesis 1:28 tells us to subdue the earth and have dominion over it. God was obviously talking to Wall Street. But then Jesus said it is harder for a rich man to enter the kingdom of heaven than for a camel to pass through the eye of a needle. But Jesus was not an entrepreneurial capitalist. If he had been, he would have started an IKEA on the shores of the Sea of Galilee.

Energy and fossil fuel companies often pay no taxes because of the extensive deductions available, like depletion allowances and the ability to defer taxes, deductions often based on laws enacted over 100 years ago—and protected by lobbyist bribery today. For a list of 60 major companies, including 30 energy companies, that paid no taxes and usually had carryover deductions see: https://itep.org/notadime/

As examples: Chevron had a U.S. income of over $5.5 billion and had a carryover loss of $142 million. Duke Energy had a U.S. income of over $3 billion and had a carryover loss of almost $650 million. So they paid no taxes. The companies extract the coal or oil and sell it to us, then they get a tax deduction for what they took and sold—a depletion allowance. What a deal! I wonder if I can get a depletion tax deduction for the grass I throw away after mowing the lawn, the leaves I rake every autumn, or the snow I shovel every winter? I guess not. If I sold it and made money on the sale I might be able to claim the tax deduction, But no! I haven't bought off any legislators to legally affirm that my grass, leaves or snow are depleted.

From 2014 to 2017 CO_2 emissions were relatively stable, but they began to rise again in 2017. And, it seems that the American government is aiding in that rise by tax breaks and subsidies to the worst polluters in the nation. Ain't capitalism wonderful? But it seems to be intent on killing its future customers!

The government could easily require that cattle feed must include bromoform ($CHBr_3$), a compound that is found in asparagopsis seaweed. 1 to 2% in the feed reduces cattle flatulence by 95 to 99%.

INTERNATIONAL EFFORTS TO REDUCE CLIMATE CHANGE UNITED NATIONS

The UN has been the major leader in this battle, but its members often become deserters when it is time to pick up a weapon! Here are some UN attempts to lead.

1987. Montreal Protocol to limit man-made aerosols that were depleting the ozone layer that filters out the harmful ultra-violet B rays that increased skin cancers. This protocol has been amended several times. It was the first UN treaty to be signed by all members.

1992. The United Nations Framework Convention on Climate Change was formed.

1997. The Kyoto Protocol was a major governmental step in recognizing and fighting global warming. The European Community and 37 industrialized countries promised to reduce greenhouse gas emissions between 2008 and 2012. The first commitment was to 5% below 1990 levels. The second commitment period was from 2013 to 2020. They agreed to reduce emissions by 18% below 1990 levels. The United States never ratified it. 100 developing countries, including China and India, were exempted. China has planted a lot of trees and built coal burning power plants to feed the trees. I don't know why our country couldn't at least have gone on a tree planting binge. Probably because trees don't produce oil—or maybe the major manufacturers can't make artificial trees that would undersell the nurseries.

2009. Copenhagen Accord. Countries pledged to limit global temperature increases to 2°C (about 3° F) over the pre-industrial level. The developed countries agreed to pay $100 billion a year by 2020 to assist poor countries affected most by climate change, including: relocating communities hit by floods and droughts and protecting water supplies. The countries agreed to provide $30 billion for three years.

Some countries refused to sign the agreement because the United States refused to cut more than 4% of its emissions by 2020. While the Republicans have a poorer record on climate change than the Democrats, both focus on the economy and rely on the financial support of their parties from the contributions of business. And who can blame them, it is certainly more important to be elected than to live!

2015-16. The Paris Climate Accord was signed by 195 countries. They pledged to cut greenhouse gas emissions by 26 to 28% below 2005 levels by 2025. They also committed $3 billion in aid for poorer countries by 2020. These countries are the most likely to suffer damage from rising sea levels and other consequences of climate change. November 4, 2016. The Paris Agreement went into force as 55 members ratified the agreement. They make up 55% of global emissions.

The Accord's goal was to keep global warming from rising more than 2° C (3.6° F) above pre-industrial levels and to work to keep the rise to under 1.5° C (2.7° F). Many experts consider that the tipping point. Beyond that, and climate change becomes unstoppable. And we know that President Trump promised to take the U.S. out of it as soon as legally possible.

Even if all countries follow the Accord, temperatures will continue to rise. The atmosphere is still reacting to the CO_2 that's already been pumped into it. Greenhouse gases have been added so quickly that temperatures haven't caught up yet.

PROGRESS AND INITIATIVES

December 12, 2017. One Planet Summit was called by French President Macron. He convened 50 world leaders to the One Planet Summit. Trump was not invited because he withdrew from the Accord. The summit focused on how to finance the global transition away from fossil fuels.

Twelve commitments were made. Emmanuel Macron warned the One Planet Summit participants: "Think long and hard, if you make a commitment, we will hold you to it." They thought long and hard... and decided to commit. These are more than commitments-- they are actions. Here they are.:

1. Responding to extreme events in island states
2. Protecting land and water against climate change
3. Mobilizing researchers and young people to work for the climate
4. Public procurement and access to green financing for local governments
5. Zero emissions target
6. Sectoral shifts towards a decarbonized economy
7. Zero pollution transport
8. Toward a carbon price compatible with the Paris Agreement

9.	Actions of central banks and businesses
10.	International mobilization of development banks
11.	Commitment by sovereign funds
12.	Mobilizing institutional investors

As an example of commitments, in number 9 'Actions of central banks and businesses" regarding how convergence can be created between the public and private-sector work for the climate? Central banks and businesses have answered the One Planet Summit's call and have committed together to take significant steps to redirect financial flows towards the low-carbon economy. 424 companies and organizations and three nations (France, UK and Sweden) support the TCFD (Task Force on Climate-related Financial Disclosures) recommendations. The commitment includes 8 out of the 10 of the largest asset managers, leading insurance companies, pension funds, and accounting organizations.

PROGRESS AND REGRESS

Global energy demand grew by 2.3 percent in 2018, nearly twice the average rate of growth since 2010, driven by a strong global economy and higher heating and cooling demand in some parts of the world. China, the United States, and India together were responsible for nearly 70 percent of the rise in the demand for energy.

In 2017, the U.S increased its GDP (the dollar value of all goods and services) by 2.2% and its CO_2 emissions increased by 2.5%. In the EU, the GDP increased 2.5%, while CO_2 emissions increased by 1.8%.

In 2018, the US increased its GDP 2.9% and had a 3.1% increase in CO_2 emissions. The European Union had a 2% increase in GDP while it decreased its CO_2 emissions by 0.7%. It should be remembered that the European Union, with its 27 countries, has a greater gross domestic product than does the United States.

PROGRESS

Europe's emissions fell by 1.3 percent and Japan's fell for the fifth year running. The European Union will cut carbon-dioxide emissions of new vehicles by 30% between 2021 and 2030. The following diagram indicates the progress of the European Union compared to the rest of the world.

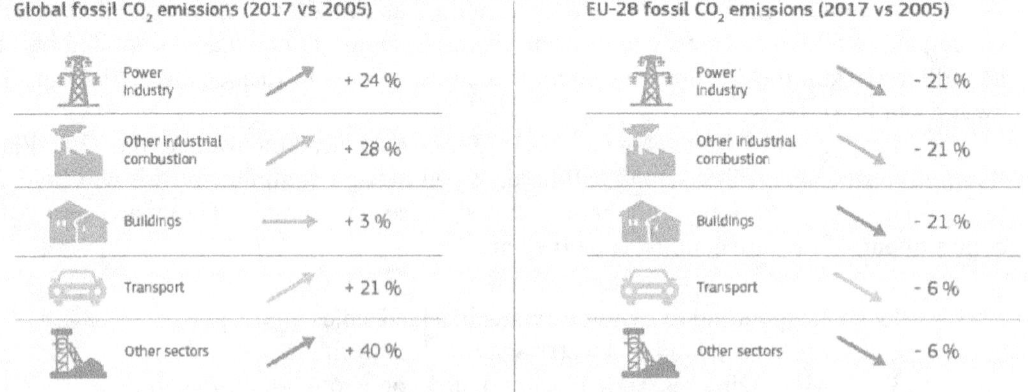

All countries should keep their commitments to pursue aggressive cuts to carbon dioxide under the Paris Agreement. Yet even if all commitments are met, global temperatures will increase between about 4.5 to 7.2 degrees Fahrenheit (2.5 to 4° C).

In May of 2018 Alaska started its own plan to stop climate change. Although it is a major oil producer, it is experiencing the effects of global warming. The permafrost is thawing, destabilizing roads, and the buildings that sit near them. Protective sea ice is melting, allowing the ocean to erode Alaskan shores. As a result, 31 coastal towns may need to relocate.

The world's 20 biggest energy corporations contribute 35% of the world's greenhouse-gas emissions. In 2017, 89% had plans to cut those emissions. But that's not enough to reach the U.N.'s target of 2 degrees Celsius. So far, 14% of the companies have goals that align with the target. Another 30% pledge do so in the next two years. Investment firms, such as HSBC Holdings and Goldman Sachs, have begun targeting more low-carbon businesses.

China produces twice as much CO_2 as the US, but has almost 4 times as many people. In 2010, China promised it would reach four climate goals by 2020.

1. Reduce CO_2 emissions by 40% below 2005 levels. (97% achieved in 2017.)
2. Increase renewable energy consumption from 9.4% to 15%. (60% achieved.)
3. Increase forest stock by 1.3 billion cubic meters. (Exceeded as of 2017.)
4. Increase forest coverage by 40 million hectares relative to 2005. (60% achieved.)

In addition, China is leading the world in electric vehicles. Almost half of the world's all-electric vehicles are sold in China. Its regulations and subsidies encourage consumers to buy them.

TAXES ON GREENHOUSE EMISSIONS

Sixty areas around the world have carbon taxes. China, Germany, Sweden, and Denmark are considering a tax on beef. Greenhouse gas emissions from livestock contribute 14.5% of the world's total.

REGRESS

The United States is responsible for 20% of the world's carbon emissions even though they have only 4.4% of the world's population.. It would be difficult for the other signatories to reach the accord's goal without U.S. participation. But they are trying.

As an American citizen, it puzzles me why Americans don't elect people who are concerned about the future of their country and the world.

About 40 to 50% of Americans vote. Where do they get the facts on which to make informed decisions?

➢ Friends and neighbors
➢ Social media—possibly influenced by Russian trolls
➢ Their political party or their representatives
➢ Impartial news sources
➢ Authoritative non-fiction books and Internet source

Emissions were up for the first time since 2015. The major reasons were increased electricity demand and the growth in trucking and aviation. In the United States' CO_2 emissions grew by 3.1 percent in 2018, reversing a decline a year earlier, while China's emissions rose by 2.5 percent and India's by 4.5 percent.

China is still building coal-fired power plants, as is India. Since 2000 the number of coal plants in the world has doubled to about 2000 gigawatts, that's 2,000,000, megawatts. To use solar power to replace these coal-fired plants it would take six and a quarter billion (6,250,000,000) photovoltaic solar panels. This would cover 12,500 square miles—about half the size of West Virginia. Meanwhile, other 550 gigawatt producing plants are being built or are planned. On the other hand, more than 225 coal-fired energy plants have been closed in the U.S. and EU.

But there is another area to be considered. Some people want to boycott decorative woods like teak and mahogany that are used in fine furniture and as walls and other appointments in homes and offices. These woods have come from the trees of the rainforest that eat so much of the air's carbon. So that sounds like a noble gesture. But often they don't consider that the wood they burn in their fireplaces not only came from CO_2 breathing trees, but burning them released the carbon back into the air. So they decry the cutting of trees in which the carbon is preserved in the wood, but applaud the burning of other trees because it may save on electricity, which may have been produced by coal. We need much more comprehensive thinking about how to most effectively conserve!

But back to Kyoto. It was predicted that by 2080 there would be an 11% decrease in rainfall for farmland in developed countries due to climate change. And 65 developing countries might lose 280 million tons of cereal production. One of the objectives was to have developed countries buy carbon emission credits from countries that had more forests and plants. That money could then be used to help underdeveloped countries develop more effective agricultural techniques and to aid them in developing bioenergy. Bioenergy is a real alternative to fossil fuels and could include fuel from animal and plant waste and alcohol developed from plants. It was hoped that by using biofuels carbon emissions could be reduced by between 5 and 25 percent of projected fossil fuel emissions for the year 2050. But it has got to become more pollution free in its development.

Then the protocol looked to developing carbon sinks, places where carbon could be stored—like forests. It also stated that the destruction of forests was responsible for a quarter of all greenhouse gases. By encouraging forest growth in undeveloped countries the polluting countries could buy credits from the people with the forests to offset the carbon they were releasing. So for example, if the U.S. was told that its carbon dioxide target was 4 billion tons by 2030 and it was putting out 5 billion tons, it could buy credits for the extra billion tons from countries with forests, like Brazil or some undeveloped country that had planted a lot of trees.

CHAPTER 8
WHERE IS THE BEST USE OF YOUR TIME

DEMONSTRATING YOUR DISPLEASURE ON THE STREETS OR KNOCKING ON DOORS TO CONVINCE VOTERS TO VOTE FOR A GREEN CANDIDATE?

Youth street protests, like those in the Arab Spring, and more recently in Lebanon and Hong Kong, sometimes get results. Adult revolutionary actions, like the American and French revolutions, had major results. But today's governments have far more firepower than any revolutionary forces can muster. So the "free India" marches of Gandhi and the "free the Blacks" marches of Martin Luther King accomplished, peacefully, the objectives of the people.

In our modern democratic republics, it is possible to re-educate or replace representatives. But since they are often in the pockets of oil producers or energy using industrialists, powerful grassroots green-advocates must use their time, and personal contact with voters, to counteract the data-mining and advertising of the opposition—those putting their profits over our lives.

With these facts and factors in mind, the deeply committed people SHOULD consider active participation in government at both the state and the national levels. If they choose not to participate personally in the functions of government, they MUST work to elect legislators by demonstrating, contributing financially, volunteering their time, and knocking on voters' doors to educate and encourage them to vote. That education must not only include the scientific facts, but also must include countering the propaganda that is certain to appear in newspapers, radio, television, Facebook and other social media. A thorough and effective program will need a group of advocates monitoring the various propaganda containing media and developing truthful and effective answers to the untruthful propaganda.

Among the actions that might be advocated:

> Pressure corporations to disclose and act on their climate-related risks.
> Require industries to buy tax credits to cover their greenhouse gas emissions.
> Eliminate tax breaks for energy companies—in fact for all companies.
> Eliminate subsidies to companies and industries that emit greenhouse gases.
> Ratify United Nations and other international protocols that deal with preventing and reversing climate change.

PRESSURING POLITICIANS

The electorate CAN, but seldom will, pressure their elected officials to do intelligent things for the citizens, rather than catering to the wishes of the elites. In the 2018 elections in the U.S. several "anti-elite" representatives were elected. Bernie Sanders in the presidential primaries of 2015-16 and 2019 and Elizabeth Warren in 2019-20 were anti-establishment candidates. Both refused to take political contributions from special interests.

In the UK, try to tax the royal family or the hundreds of dukes and barons out of their riches and land holdings—land given four or five hundred years ago by King "what's his name."

The elites are the leaders in: business, labor, religions, government, royal families, and the military. They have the power to influence people with their words and actions. They can buy radio and television stations, put ads or propaganda on YouTube or Facebook, or use troll accounts like Russia and other countries, and many people, have done. They can influence us to vote, or not to vote, through any of the many data-mining programs.

When the UK is 23rd and the U.S. is 31st on the international PISA scores for educational achievement (behind: China and Singapore) you can understand how easy it is to hoodwink us—the supposedly superior Anglos.

PRESSURING GOVERNMENTS TO CURB THE EXCESSES

Since national economies and personal tax increases are the major impediments to effective climate change, maybe they should be the targets for significant reductions in greenhouse gas emissions. And, REMEMBER, reduction of greenhouse gases will be painful for all of us.

➢ Driving your car should be much more expensive.

➢ Solar, wind and tidal power will cost much more to install for individuals and industries—but will be cheaper in the long run.

➢ Governments could make laws to forbid trading with countries who are not meeting the goals set by the most recent scientific findings for a realistic and meaningful reduction in greenhouse gases and a drastic cut in fossil fuel use.

➢ Or apply very high tariffs to goods and services sold by countries that are not meeting realistic goals in reducing greenhouse gases.

➢ Overpopulation must be quickly reversed, preferably voluntarily rather than through starvation, drowning, terrorism or war.

➢ Richer countries might pay people to be sterilized—so that the action is voluntary.

The costs will have to borne by you, the consumer. Although pressure might be brought, through changing corporate stock-purchasing options, reducing stockholder payouts and reducing CEO salaries. Such an economic onslaught would require a major overhaul of the self-centered thinking of most of us and our leaders.

➢ The price to save the planet will be high—it is, after all, a large planet.

➢ Realistically, we can pray—but the responsibility is ours.

➢ We can complain and demonstrate—but we must physically DO! What else can we do?

➢ Require industries to buy tax credits to cover their greenhouse gas emissions.

➢ Pressure corporations to disclose and act on their climate-related risks. 100 companies are responsible for more than 70% of greenhouse gas emissions. The worst are ExxonMobil, Shell, BP, and Chevron. These four companies contribute 6.49% alone.

➢ Require individuals to buy tax credits for their own emissions---gasoline and utility taxes could handle much of this.

➢ Vote for candidates who promise a solution to climate change. The <u>Sunrise Movement</u> is pressuring candidates to adopt a <u>Green New Deal</u>. There are <u>500 candidates</u> who have vowed not to accept campaign contributions from the oil industry.

CHAPTER 9
CARBON SINKS

Ultimately, trees of any shape, size, or genetic origin help absorb CO_2. Most scientists agree that the least expensive and perhaps the easiest way for individuals to help offset the CO_2 that they generate in their everyday lives is to plant a tree...any tree, as long as it is appropriate for the given region and climate.

Those who wish to help larger tree planting efforts can donate money or time to the National Arbor Day Foundation or American Forests in the U.S., or to the Tree Canada Foundation in Canada.

But it depends on such things as the number of trees and other plants in the world and how much more CO_2 the ocean can absorb. It has been absorbing about half of the human produced CO_2 up to now. But as the ocean warms the CO_2 is held closer to the surface and the amount of gas that can be absorbed by the whole ocean is reduced.

Then there is the fact that when the climate warms, the plants don't absorb as much carbon dioxide, probably because they reduce their growing rate so that they can conserve water. So, CO_2 emissions are not being handled as well as they were a hundred years ago. But there's more to the mix. As the world warms, there is some evidence that the tree line is rising in the northern latitudes and in the higher altitudes. But then there are some other negatives, like tree damaging insects that increase as the climate warms. The average temperature is expected to increase by almost one and a half degrees Celsius by 2050. It may not sound like much but on a global scale it is immense. If we do nothing, the Earth's temperature will probably rise 4 degrees Celsius this century.

CREATE SINKS

Sinks may be long or short term possibilities; For example, if you plant a tree it will help for the life of the tree. But, when it dies or is burned for cooking or for a decorative cozy atmosphere, the carbon it had captured is released to the atmosphere it once called home!

TREES TO FIGHT CLIMATE CHANGE

Dave Nowak, a researcher at the U.S. Forest Service's Northern Research Station in Syracuse, New York, has studied the use of trees for carbon sequestration in urban settings across the United States. A 2002 study he co-authored lists the common horse-chestnut, Douglas fir, black walnut, American sweetgum, ponderosa pine, red pine, white pine, London plane, Hispaniolan pine, scarlet oak, red oak, Virginia live oak, and bald cypress as examples of trees especially good at absorbing and storing CO_2. Avoid planting trees that require a lot of maintenance, since the burning of fossil fuels used to power trucks and chainsaws cuts into the net effectiveness of the tree's total effectiveness. A ten year old eucalyptus or pine tree would sequester about 70 pounds of carbon dioxide in a year.

A trillion trees can be planted on the 1.7 billion hectares (4.2 billion acres or 6.5 million square miles—an area the size of the U.S. and China) that are available and not being used for agriculture.

Anyway!, chopping down that fir tree for your traditional holiday decoration has some negative consequences for your children and grandchildren. Maybe you should leave a bottle of oxygen in their Christmas stocking!

CHAPTER 10
OVERPOPULATION—THE ELEPHANT IN THE ROOM

DON'T READ THESE NEXT TWO CHAPTERS IF YOU ARE BOUND BY TRADITIONS

OVERPOPULATION—THE MAJOR FACTOR IN CLIMATE CHANGE

These are very long chapters that merely scratch the surface of the many problems related to our present state of overpopulation and to the number of problems that will occur if the number of people are reduced to a sustainable population level. The suggested level is less than 2 billion according to Dr. David Pimentel, Professor Emeritus of Cornell University, probably the world's foremost authority on the issue. The 2 million number assumes that all people on the planet will live at the standards that the West enjoys.

As in any area where suggestions are made, the possibilities must be explored. It is not enough to cay "cut carbon dioxide emissions," we must suggest how it can be done most effectively and with the least disruption to the society. Reducing the population has many negatives, such as: religious objections, the economic interests of manufacturers for an ever-increasing customer-base, and the government's professed need for more soldiers—even though the next big war will be fought with drones, missiles and atomic bombs. But no need to worry, as Albert Einstein told us—the war after the next one will be fought with sticks and stones. And we might add, that if we don't thin out our populations voluntarily, that next war will do it for us. But do we really want another "war to end all wars?" We had two in the last century and we still have some world leaders rattling their atomic sabers.

We see today, the combination of:
- Too many people for a family or nation to support,
- Too few people educated to the level necessary in today's technological society,
- Too many migrants fleeing their environs from poverty and war,
- Too many migrant freeing to opportunity,
- Empathy for the migrants who didn't choose their birth situations,
- Reduction of empathy as an excess of migrants disrupt the accepting societies (economic costs, religious and social class differences,--and often: job losses of the native born and the possibility of increased criminality)

Many believe that the increase in the dissatisfied among us should be stopped at the source, preventing their births rather than asking other countries to welcome them after they are grown. Poland is a case in point. With more than 38 million people, who are aging, they need more people to pay for the increasing number of retirees. But with a native-born population of 97%, they certainly don't want non-Polish immigrants—although over 1.2 million Poles have left their country for greener employment pastures. So they closed their borders to people who want in, but open them for people who want out. Men retire at 65 so need 12 years of pension. Women retire at 60 so need 20 years of pension.

How should they solve their problems? Raise retirement ages? No! Bring in immigrant workers? No! Encourage more births? Yes! They have done this by giving $135 per child from the second child (for the first child for poor mothers), and a minimum retirement for mothers of four. Thank you Poland, for your efforts to increase climate change.

In the Southern Hemisphere, Sub-Saharan Africa has reduced birthrates from 6.7 per woman in 1985 to 4.8 today—but that is still more than the world or the family needs today. Somalia at 6.2 and Mali at 6.0 are a shade higher than Mauritius at 1.4 and South Africa at 2.4. But don't worry, Europe will take the excess!

Whoops! Many in Europe now oppose taking in immigrants. Poland and Hungary have erected walls. A recent poll in 2018, found that majorities in all seven polled countries were opposed to accepting more migrants: Germany (72%), Denmark (65%), Finland (64%), Sweden (60%), United Kingdom (58%), France (58%) and Norway (52%). So empathy is waning. Will the overpopulated countries attempt to curb births? Will the world assist them? Or will our age-old traditions continue to bless parenthood while the increased population curses the planet?

OUR TRADITIONS ARE THE HURDLES IMPEDING OUR PROGRESS

When we talk about overcoming traditions, it is extremely difficult. Whether you are having to take public transportation rather than drive your car, stop burning wood in your fireplace, using plastic Christmas trees instead of the carbon-catching millions of fir trees we have traditionally killed every winter to celebrate the birth of Light and the advent of Armageddon. Or, what about refraining from using your home electrical system, when the electricity comes from burning fossil fuels--it is disconcerting, if not downright troublesome. But these nuisances are minuscule when we compare them with reducing population--not having a child that you want. This can be a major impediment to reversing climate change--but it is THE major one! It is the elephant in the room that nobody wants to see!

Great thinkers have suggested utopias that would challenge our lethargy. Rousseau would have us return to the mythical days of the noble savages—to equality. Plato gave us the blueprint for the ideal method of being governed—but we continually reject the ideal. History is clear that to thin out our population we need a great war and a great warrior—a Caesar, a Tamerlane, a Napoleon, or a Tojo. Swords and spears, or bullets and bombs, are the guillotines of our hopes and prayers.

Will collective intelligence ever override the flow of fear and the whimper of hope that have pulled our human race to the brink of Niagara?

CAN WE SLAY THE TYRANTISAURUS OF TRADITION—AND SAVE OURSELVES?

If we encourage or require people to reduce their family size, we run afoul of many religions and our species-long requirement for preservation by reproduction. Tribes or countries with more young men become formidable adversaries. Warriors have always been a necessity. As trade, and lots of lots of manufacturing, became the marks of a successful country, consumers were needed. In the more primitive areas of our world, and sometimes in the developed world, the man or woman with many children could point to his or her fecundity as a mark of their superiority.

China's "one child" policy is continually bashed for three reasons:
1.   It impeded people's freedom,
2.   Abortions of female fetuses has resulted in 30 million more males, and,

3.   More workers are needed to support China's greying population.

These are true, but they don't tell the whole story. The 400 million fewer children born allowed for the elimination of poverty in the country, better education for all, the funding of economic infrastructure, the significant increase in living standards, and the number of millionaires and billionaires.

The World Bank set the international poverty line at $1.90 per day in 2015, but each country sets its own standards for poverty. In the U.S. it is $32 a day for a single person under 65 and $67 a day for a family of four. The CIA World Factbook for 2018 lists: China with 2.7% living in poverty, the U.S. with 15.1%, the UK with 15%, Haiti with 59%, Zimbabwe 72.3%, and war-torn Syria with 82.5% of its population in poverty.

On the other end of the economic scale, China is second to the U.S. in the number of billionaires—285 to 705. (Compare to Germany with 146, Russia 102, and UK with 97.) Also, of October 2019, there were more Chinese than Americans in the world's richest 10%. The average (mean) incomes (total earnings divided by the number of income earners) are deceptive because the millionaire and billionaire incomes raise the average. A more accurate picture would be seen by looking at the median income—the income of the earner at the exact middle of all earners.

Per capita incomes	1980	2018	% Increase
United States	$48,400	$62,800	23%
United Kingdom	$39,400	$43,400	9%
China	$4,500	$9,770	117%
World	$9,500	$11,300	16%

The obvious point is—if a rapid increase of income, and what it can do for increasing one's ability to acquire higher education and/or travel extensively, increases one's freedom, reducing population is a very positive factor in freedom. With the average cost of raising a child to age 21 in the United Kingdom of 273,000 British pounds ($358,000) and $233,000 to raise a child in the U.S.to age 18, plus expenses for college for the next few years –you can see the financial freedom advantages to having fewer children.

IT IMPEDED PEOPLE'S FREEDOM

According to the World Bank, more than 850 million Chinese people have been lifted out of extreme poverty. We might assume that poverty somewhat affects peoples' freedom! Am I wrong, here? China's poverty rate fell from 88 percent of its population in 1981 to 0.7 percent in 2015.

Then there is their progress in developing university educational opportunities. In 2002, there were about 2000 higher education institutions in the People's Republic of China. Today there are 3,000 and three are rated in the top 100 in the world. More than 28 million students are currently studying in them, this is the same number as in the U.S.. Additionally, last year 662,000 Chinese students left China to study at overseas universities. This was about 70,000 more than the year before. Most return home with new knowledge and ideas.

China is doing quite well in producing STEM (science, technology, engineering, mathematics) graduates. Only Russia and Iran produce more technical graduates as a percentage of their populations—and they were both well ahead of China in 1980, when the "one child" policy was implemented.

STEM graduates

Country	Population in millions	STEM graduates per million	% of population
China	1,433	4,700	3.2
India	1,56	2,600	1.9
US	330	568	1.7
Russia	146	561	3.8
Iran	83	335	4.0
Indonesia	270	206	0.7
Japan	126	195	1.5

Those of us who regularly attend scientific conferences can attest to the unbelievable advancement of Chinese science. When Chinese scientists presented their work from about 1990 to 2000, we smiled. They were discovering things with the same instruments that we in the West had discovered in the 1950s. But by 2010 they were state of the art. Their scientific instruments and their knowledge of their scientific fields had leap-frogged over the decades. The increased money available, since they didn't have to educate and care for 400 million children, became available to send their students to the best universities in the world and to finance their rapid economic development.

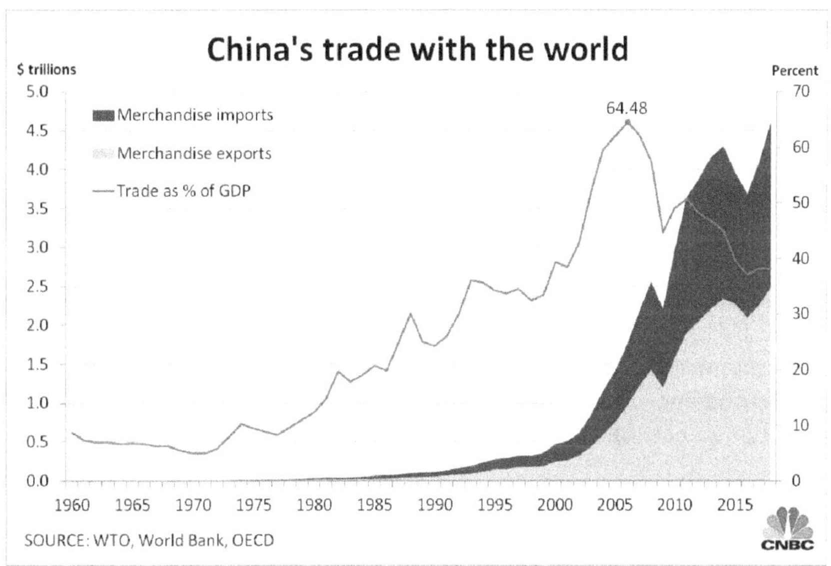

Does this sound like the Chinese people's freedom was impeded a great deal because some of them could not have more than one baby?

ABORTIONS OF FEMALE FETUSES HAS RESULTED IN 30 MILLION MORE MALES

This is true, but it is a result of an antiquated family tradition—not of the one child policy. Males were supposed to be better able to support their aging parents—but that was before women were allowed to attend the universities and enter the workforce in highly paid jobs. The long-held idea that women should be barefoot and pregnant in the kitchen has been submerged with the blessings of contraception and safe abortions that have allowed women the same opportunities as men.

In the U.S. 56% of university students are female. In China it is 52.5%. Females are also in the majority in the UK and many other countries. So if taking care of aging parents financially is important, women will be able to do it better.

MORE WORKERS ARE NEEDED TO SUPPORT CHINA'S GREYING POPULATION.

This is a concern in many countries. Short-sighted vote-hungry politicians have assumed that there will always be 5 or 6 workers paying into their inadequate pension funds to pay for the retirees who were never required to contribute enough to pay for their pensions.

If we continue to increase the population, with 5 to 7 new workers to pay for the older workers, we will need geometrically more workers every generation. So if we need five more workers now to support each retiree, in 20 to 40 years we will need 25, Then 40 more years 125 workers to support the 25 of the last generation. All this while the number of employees needed is reducing because of robotics, computerization, 3D printing, and artificial intelligence.

If we calculate the number of people needed to support every worker in retirement, and if only half of today's population of 7,500,000,000 works and we need five workers to support each retiree, in forty years we will need 18.5 billion workers. Then forty years later we will need 90 billion workers. It wouldn't be too long before we would need a population of a trillion people. But that will never happen because floods, famines and hurricanes will wipe out a large number of us. Our politicians seem to keep getting us deeper and deeper into the quicksand of our own genocide. But it really doesn't matter as long as they keep getting elected. In fact, if we elect the appropriate people, they will assure us that climate change doesn't exist and that any abortion is terribly wrong. Certainly, the world needs more children—especially those who are not wanted.

RETIREMENT AGES

American retirement age has increased only two years in the last 80.

In the US when Social Security was enacted, the retirement age was 65 and the average lifespan was 64. We have recently raised the retirement age to 67, for those born since 1960, but our lifespans are in the early 80s—and increasing.

In the U.S., our retirement contributions are generally used up by our early 70s. The government must then make up for our lack of adequate contributions for 5 to 10 more years of our retirement.

As I remember, one of those messages carved in stone on Mount Sinai was that we should be able to retire at age 65. Most blasphemous countries allow it to be between 55 and 60. I hope there's enough oil under their workplaces to support 30 years of retirement!

China recently increased the number of children allowed per family to two. There were several reasons for this. One of which was to provide a workforce to support the aging population.

Lifespans in China have increased from 35 years in 1948 to 66 years in 1976 to 76 years today. Retirement age is between 50 and 55 for women and 6o for men. How much will today's young workers need to contribute for their extra 15 to 20 years of retirement?

The retirement age in China currently is 60 for men and 55 for female civil servants and 50 for female workers. By 2038 there will be an equal retirement age for women and men set at 67. (Women's retirement age will reach 65 in 2030 and 67 in 2038).

Tradition continually blocks our thinking about issues. For China, rather than having more children, they might raise the age of retirement to 68 or 70 for both men and women. Of course, the people will object and possibly rebel. Look at what happened in Russia and France in 2019 when their presidents attempted to tackle tradition and inch closer to a realistic pension plan. Demonstrations and riots erupted. So don't mess with traditions—no matter how antiquated and harmful to society they are. Astute politicians will always give the electorate what they want. Let their children pay for it in taxes or in a national bankruptcy.

ENOUGH OF CHINA—HOW ABOUT THE REST OF US?

With Pope Francis condemning atomic war, but encouraging more children to be born, is he seeing the whole picture? Do ExxonMobil and Koch Industries, going after profits today, realize that their future consumers will be significantly reduced with the growing specter of mass annihilation? Do the Mormons, seeking to free the infinite number of souls that were created when God started us on our fateful path, understand that the present surge of souls will be reduced to a trickle? Reducing the number born now will result in more available souls to save than would be available if we experience a catastrophic series of population reducing calamities--like mass famines and gigantic storms.

A GLANCE AT PEOPLE AND POLLUTION

The most emissions from fossil fuels come from China and the United States. In terms of CO_2 emissions *per capita* per year, China is ranked only 47th, at 7.5 metric tons per capita. The US is ranked 11th at 16.5 tons per capita. India is the third highest country in terms of absolute emissions, but only 158th in terms of per capita output with 1.7 metric tons per capita.

Australia has an average per capita footprint of 17 tons, and Canada has 15.6 tons per capita. So reducing population in the U.S., Canada or Australia by one person will be about the same as reducing 150 to 200 people in Somalia or Eritrea in terms of fossil fuel use!

Wait a minute! In much of southern Africa, especially east Africa, there are some big problems. CO_2 absorbing forests are being reduced significantly. This is done for firewood and charcoal production. So Africa is a problem too.

The United Nations' IPCC estimates that about 15% of carbon dioxide is emitted from wood-burning for cooking fires in Africa. There are about 2.1 billion people in Africa living below the poverty line.

In countries in East Africa, such as in Somalia, Zambia, and Madagascar, charcoal is produced for sale to other African countries for cooking, to Arab countries for hookka smoking, and world-wide for barbeque cooking. This charcoal production is usually done illegally on government lands—and is illegal according to the United Nations. The trees that are chopped down are not replaced. Obviously then, the wood is burned—releasing its carbon onto the atmosphere and carbon-capturing trees are lost in the process.

In the last six years in Somalia, 8.2 million trees have been removed. In Uganda the forest cover has been reduced in the last 15 years from 24% to 9%. So Africa's contribution to greenhouse gas production is not reflected in the charts we see of the greenhouse gases that are produced from burning fossil fuels—like coal, oil, gasoline, other gases and from permafrost thawing.

Somalia makes about half of the African profits from total charcoal sales of $360 million a year. The al Qaeda linked al Shabab takes about 10% of this profit as protection money, which it uses to fund its terrorist activities. So we have another unexpected villain on our highway to survival!

Across Africa the charcoal trade is destroying the forest cover which has been absorbing the CO_2 emissions from cooking fires and from industry. The European Space Agency has found that biomass (ie. wood, manure) burning is responsible for about 30% of climate changing greenhouse gases. Congo has the second largest forest in the world—

after the Amazon. The increasing population needs more jobs and more cooking charcoal—so the forest and the world suffer.

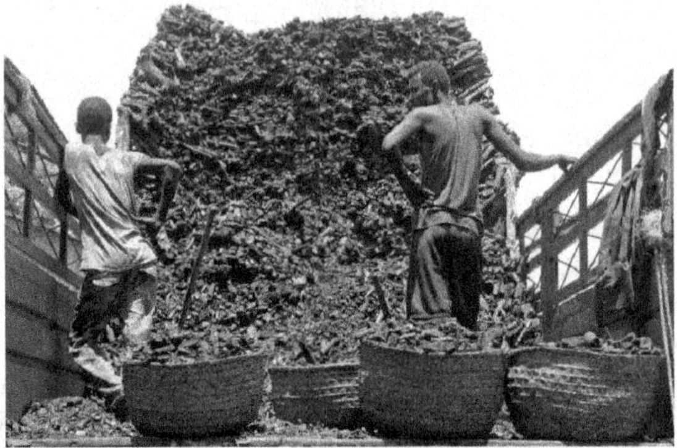

Truck full of charcoal in Somalia

You can imagine that burning over a million trees a year is adding to the greenhouse effect caused by the carbon dioxide released. So rich and poor people are contributing to the warming--yes, the rich are worse, but we are all a part of the problem.

We know that there is a strong relationship between income and per capita fossil fuel CO_2 emissions. But Europe is doing a far better job than other major polluting countries. The global average of carbon dioxide emissions is about 4.8 tons per person. Some European countries have emissions not far from the global average: Portugal is about 5.3 tons and France and the UK are just a bit higher than Portugal—because they are producing much of their energy from renewable and nuclear sources. But China's CO_2 emissions per capita have more than tripled in the past 15 years.

HIGHEST TOTAL CO_2 EMISSIONS BY COUNTRY IN KILO-TONS (THOUSANDS OF TONS)

1	China	10,291,926
2	United States	5,254,279
3	India	2,238,377
4	Russia	1,705,345
5	Japan	1,214,048
6	Germany	719,883
7	Iran.	649,480
8	Saudi Arabia	601,046
9	Korea, Rep.	587,156
10	Canada	537,193
11	Brazil	529,808
12	South Africa	489,771
13	Mexico	480,270
14	Indonesia	464,176

15	United Kingdom	419,820
16	Australia	361,261
17	Turkey	345,981
18	Italy	320,411

LOWEST CO₂ EMISSIONS PER CAPITA

By comparison, some of the poorest countries produce practically zero CO_2 from fossil fuel emissions per capita

Eritrea	0.089
Niger	0.089
Malawi	0.083
Ethiopia	0.075
Somalia	0.063
Central African Republic	0.061
Chad	0.040
Burundi	0.033
Lesotho	0.009

You are already protesting against removing many of the benefits that our economic system and our technological pampering has given us--undreamed of comforts and conveniences. We no longer have to walk great distances to talk to a friend. We don't have to send smoke signals either. We can e-mail, Skype, Facetime, Facebook, WhatsApp or even drive to see each other. We don't have to work 10 or 12 hours a day, 6 or 7 days a week, to make a living. There are more ways to kill a night than just playing cards. We had radio, then television, the Internet—and now video games. Life keeps getting easier, with more free time and more enjoyable ways to spend it. How come? More fossil fuel is available for our transportation needs. There is more electrical power for our air conditioning, heating, TVs, and for research to make life even easier.

So, our long-held traditions, and even our recently acquired traditions, must be adjusted as climate change heats our air, increases the intensity of our storms, and makes forest fires more likely and more damaging.

We must expect more atmospheric problems to darken our days—both heat and cold as well as wet and dry. Our taxes will rise.

INCREASED TAXES OR NATIONAL DEBT

Our national debts will increase—if we can still find people to lend to us! We may even find it necessary to change our economic system. Governments rely on two or three sources for the money that fuels them.

➞   Taxes

➞   Borrowing, and

➞   Government ownership of part or all of some industries. American politicians call socialism (government ownership of all or part of the industries) totally unacceptable. The U.S. relies on the first two ways to finance itself, although it does own the Postal System, the Tennessee Valley Authority, mortgage and loan companies (Freddie Mac, Fannie May) and a number of other businesses. So the United States is partially socialistic. Not as much as most modern countries, which may be one of the reasons that the U.S. is only 18th on the UN international happiness scale. (For more on this read: "Make America Great Again—Like Norway.")

Except for Bernie Sanders, Americans decry socialism. Few see that their sacred Social Security System is communistic ("as Karl Marx wrote, "From each according to his ability to each according to his needs."). Medicaid is equally communistic, being based on need. Medicare is more socialistic since it only covers those who paid in. (Lenin said that "Socialism is from each according to his ability, to each according to his work.") Even the government-paid educational systems, which are becoming more common around the world, can be considered to be communistic since they are available to all for a certain number of years.

So our anti-communist and anti-socialist traditions are overlooked when something, we see as good, sneaks into our capitalist global view. The U.S. didn't have Social Security until the mid-30s. Thirty years later President Lyndon Johnson began the enactment of laws that eventually led to Medicaid and Medicare—and more traditions were absorbed into the abyss of tradition.

What next?—Eu-genics (reducing potential genetic or epigenetic problems, such as genes related to violence, psychosis, low intelligence, etc.), eu-parenting (parent licensing—to ascertain potential parent's abilities and aptitudes for financial and psychological caretaking), required sterilization, voluntary sterilization, taxing children, etc. Or should we allow, or encourage, the unrestricted increase of population.

The reality of unrestricted family size will certainly increase ecological problems such as: decrease of natural resources, decreasing fresh water available, increasing air and water pollution, increased greenhouse gases, increasing northward and westward migration, with the strong possibility of more wars (water-wars and wars for more territory), and more terrorism.

There are too many people in the world. Some of them are very good for the world as scientists, some legislators, creative entrepreneurs, artists, etc. Some are very bad for the world, like: warlords, terrorists, criminals, and abusers of different sorts. we might even add here those who cannot contribute to the society because of inherited inabilities.

Of course, if we begin to eliminate potential citizens, we run the risk of criticism from religions and other groups. For example, if we were to attempt to instigate a family-planning program in Mali, Nicaragua, or India, we would probably be accused of genocide. But then, if we don't thin out the population, we are all potential victims of genocide. So do we want our greenhouse gases to kill or inconvenience most of the population of the world, or do we aid in lowering the fertility rate in some areas while we improve their educational opportunities and their chances for happiness. The United Nations happiness scale does not list those countries with high fertility rates in the same high categories as those with lower fertility rates.

When we look at some of the high fertility rate countries, we often see children being sold into slavery or released into the overpopulated cities without parents. CNN recently aired a program, originating in Africa, where boys as young as four had been given to a supposedly religious man who ran schools. The boys were released every morning with buckets to beg for money or hopefully they would find jobs. They were given quotas of money they had to bring back to the adults. They slept in the open-air in slums. Is this what you would want for your children?

When we look at eugenics, people will say that that is what Hitler did. One should not criticize an idea because of the person who advocated it, rather than for the idea being expressed, this is called a logical fallacy. In fact, it is called the *ad hominem* fallacy. The fact is that Hitler loved his mother intensely. He said she was the most important person in his life. Should we therefore criticize all people who love their mothers? In the United States a number of years ago, eugenics was used to stop the reproduction of some African-Americans.

Hitler's plan was to eliminate those who he thought were inferior: the Jews, the Slavs, homosexuals, and the physically or mentally handicapped. But he also had a plan to increase the number of people in the higher "master race." So he encouraged the high level men to father with a high level women.

CHAPTER 11
WHAT ARE SOME OPTIONS TO REDUCE POPULATION?

We will look at some options for reducing population—but it is not enough to say that we must do something, we must look deeper at the hows and the whys. For example, it is not enough to tell Poland that they must immediately stop burning coal. 80% of its electricity is generated from the work of the 100,000 coal miners. The economics of Poland is a major concern for them. The survival of the planet's population is a concern for the rest of us. It is the narrowly viewed NOW versus the future of humanity. How do we solve the problem?

In the concern for overpopulation, we have the same "now verses the future" problem. We will suggest some guidelines for the population of the future, but people won't like the possibilities. They flaunt tradition! But they need to be outlined if we are going to attempt to survive—and survive in a cooperative and more peaceful world.

So here goes!—Some ideas for reducing and improving the society that is threatening their home!

VOLUNTARY

These options may need financial assistance from richer countries to poorer countries.

> ➢ Abortion on demand.
> ➢ Euthanasia on demand. This could include not only sick people, but others who wish to die. There are about 800,000 suicides in the world annually, 47,000 in the U.S.
> ➢ Contraceptives on demand.
> ➢ Sterilizations on demand.
> ➢ Enticement to voluntary sterilization by monetary awards from governments or private sources.

MANDATORY AND SEVERE

One option is to do nothing now, but to let Nature takes its course as the warming climate increases violent storms, larger forest fires, and more extensive famines—and possibly more wars and terrorism as various physical and social stresses lead to violence. More migration is already happening. Water wars and the closing of borders to immigrants are strong possibilities—both have happened in the past.

We are all going to die—that is determined when we are born. Is it imperative to do all things possible to protect and extend every life? Should mass shooters, when found guilty, languish in taxpayer paid prisons while they contribute to global warming after causing the deaths of productive and innocent people? Should Hitler or Attila or John Wilkes Booth have been drowned at birth? Should there be any criteria to live freely? We now have severe penalties for murderers—even death in many countries!

Are all lives equal? Are all lives equally valuable—even when they are anti-social? Even though they do not contribute to the society? Even if they are terminally ill? If so, we might consider some other options, even if they run counter to UN and EU rights.

> ➢ One option would be to have national or international lotteries that would allow the lucky winners to have a child. The recent United Nations and European

Union protocols for treating everyone equally might approve of this—except that those who didn't win, were not treated equally.

- China's recent "one child policy" treated people equally, but restricted the liberty of those who wanted more children. The radical reduction in family size –from a fertility rate of 3.81 in 1975 to 1.7 today—will not be realized as a downturn in their population until about 2050. The 70 year lag, from the introduction of the program until a population reduction is realized, is too long a period to have the immediate effect we need today.
- Increased capital punishment with speedier appeals and executions—possibly increasing capital crimes to: rape, child molestation, illegal drug sellers, and maybe even tax evaders and burglars!
- People who choose to use dangerous drugs, then overdose, could be left to die. Many are not contributing to the society—and they bring in more criminal suppliers.
- As the importance of genetics became known, "eugenics" has been considered and used. The equalitarian emphasis of today's politics makes it a long-shot option. But it will be discussed below.
- Eu-parenting, while never used, has been suggested with varying parental qualities and abilities being the necessities for parent licensing. The equalitarian bent of democratic thinking makes this option another long-shot. While legally all children belong to the state, it nearly always lets the natural or adoptive parents raise them—even when the children are abused or neglected. It will also be discussed below.

Attempts to reduce populations in India, Africa, Brazil or Boston will elicit cries of "genocide," while producing more polluters is somehow praiseworthy! Just look at the religious accolades afforded to the Duggar family with their 19 children. A reality TV show contract and lots of positive publicity was their reward. The last I heard there were nine grandchildren for this ever-expanding family. But if we only look a little deeper, we see that their neighbors had to pay taxes to put these children through school—about $3,600,000. Then there is the carbon footprint, of every child, of 20 metric tons of carbon dioxide per year. That is about 400 metric tons per year for the family, and if each lives to be about 80 years old, it will be about 32,000 metric tons of carbon dioxide for each person—or about 640,000 metric tons during the lives of the immediate family. So the Duggar family, not counting the grandchildren, has a carbon footprint equivalent to 87 American cars each driven 12,000 miles per year. So, "yea!" for the family that was fruitful and multiplied! But then there is the carbon footprint of each child and their children, and their children—if the world survives!

These good Baptists followed their holy book—where it tells us in Genesis 1:28 to ". . . Be fruitful and multiply." But they might have read the whole verse:

"And God blessed them, and God said unto them, Be fruitful, and multiply, and replenish the earth, and subdue it: and have dominion over the fish of the sea, and over the fowl of the air, and over every living thing that moveth upon the earth."

It seems that the earth is more "replenished" than it has ever been. And certainly, the descendants of Adam and Eve have not subdued it. In fact, the earth now seems to be subduing those descendants! And what about all of us living things that moveth upon the earth? We have done a terrible job of dominating us and our world!

TOO MANY PEOPLE USING TOO MUCH FOSSIL FUEL!

There are too many people in the world. Some of them are very good for the world as scientists, effective legislators, creative entrepreneurs, some artists, etc. Some are very bad for the world, like: warlords, terrorists, criminals, and abusers of different sorts. We might even add here, those who cannot contribute to the society because of inherited inabilities.

GENOCIDE

Of course, if we begin to eliminate potential citizens, we run the risk of criticism from religions and other groups. For example, if we were to attempt to instigate a family-planning program in Mali, Nicaragua, or India, we would probably be accused of genocide. But then, if we don't thin out our population, we are all potential victims of genocide. So, do we want our greenhouse gases to kill or inconvenience most of the population of the world or do we aid in lowering the fertility rate in some areas while we improve their educational opportunities and their chances for happiness. The United Nations happiness scale does not list any of those countries with high fertility rates in the same high categories as those with lower fertility rates.

When we look at some of the high fertility rate countries, we often see children being sold into slavery or released into the overpopulated cities without parents. CNN recently aired a program, originating in Africa, where boys as young as four have been given to supposedly religious man who ran schools. The boys were released every morning with buckets to beg or hopefully to find jobs. They were given quotas of money they had to bring back to the adults. They slept in the open-air in slums. Is this what you would want for your children?

Generally, the more children a family has the lower their happiness level. (For those interested in seeing more details on this, we suggest reading "A Global Perspective on Happiness and Fertility" by Rachel MaRgolis and Mikko MyRskylä at: https://www.ncbi.nlm.nih.gov/pmc/articles/PMC3345518/

THE BIG QUESTIONS

The first question is—Shall we attempt to limit population?

The second is--should we try to control the types of people, since modern life seems to need more intelligent and more loving people. Math and science aptitudes and training, not manual labor are needed—and even more important, people who are loving and not intent on shooting, raping and robbing us. How can we do these things? Do we want to?

If we want to raise the intelligence level of the population, and possibly change a tendency for other elements of personality—like violence, lack of impulse control, and sexuality—we have some knowledge about how to do this. For this we must look at eugenics and epigenetics. For developing a well-balanced person with the ability to love, parenting is essential—and eugenics may also play a role.

INFANTICIDE

We could just kill unwanted babies. But this idea is generally frowned on in today's more advanced cultures. However, it has been practiced since prehistoric times. Many Neolithic sites have been unearthed confirming this practice.. It is clear that family sizes had to be controlled because there was not enough food for the family or tribe. In many later cultures, child sacrifice to the gods became common. It has been found throughout the Middle Ages, and we see it today in many societies, including our own. How often have you heard of a young woman leaving her newborn in a dumpster?

We know that it was quite common in ancient Greece and Rome—in fact the mythological founders of Rome, Romulus and Remus, had been thrown in the Tiber River before being rescued and raised by a wolf.

Primitive tribes and cultures, as well as the destitute or unwilling today, have unburdened themselves of surplus infants. While the Abrahamic religions of Judaism.

Christianity and Islam have generally opposed infanticide, Christians have often opted for a more comfortable life here and now, rather than waiting for the hereafter with a large brood of starving children huddled in cramped corners. 19th century England records many illegal infanticides and the hanging of many murderous mothers.

EUGENICS

Modern eugenic ideas have been around as long as genetics has been studied. Sir Francis Galton, a major mid-19th Century scientific genius, coined the term "eugenics." He was a highly regarded scientist and mathematician. His forays into science and his extensive traveling opened many doors. He invented the concept of correlation as well as coining the word "eugenics" and the term "nature versus nurture." He pioneered the field of behavioral genetics with his "twin" studies-- researching whether identical twins raised in different environments would be different and whether fraternal twins raised in the same environment would be similar. His observations led him to believe in both eugenics and in equality of opportunity-- by increasing inheritance taxes to form a tax base for supporting genetically gifted poorer people to be able to have more superior children.

As previously mentioned, people will say that eugenics is a bad idea because Hitler advocated eugenics. But, one should not criticize an idea because of the person who advocated it, rather than for the idea being expressed.

The fact is that Hitler's ideas followed those of American and German scientists. California led the way in sterilizing unfit people in the early 1900s. In the 1930s Hitler continued with such sterilizations, then with gas chambers. (That was certainly extreme!) He also required people who planned to marry to undergo testing to uncover any tendency to hereditary diseases.

Hitler's idea was to eliminate: the Jews, who were religiously and racially inferior, the Slavs who were racially inferior. He also wanted to get rid of the homosexuals and physically and mentally inferior people, who were usually institutionalized in state or private facilities—because they were not normal and stood in the way of his development of his "master race" development plans.

Eugenics was also supported by African-American intellectuals such as W. E. B. Du Bois and many academics at the traditionally black colleges: Tuskegee University, Howard University, and Hampton University. They believed that the best blacks were as good as the best whites and that "The Talented Tenth" of all races should mix. Du Bois believed "only fit blacks should procreate to eradicate the race's heritage of moral iniquity."

In Michigan a compulsory sterilization bill was introduced in 1897, but was not passed. In 1905 Pennsylvania passed a sterilization bill, but it was vetoed by the governor. Two years later Indiana passed such a eugenic law. Several states quickly followed. The U.S. Supreme Court, in 1927, allowed for sterilization for some patients in a home for the mentally retarded in Virginia. Fifteen years later it disallowed the sterilization of prisoners. From 1910 and for 50 years there were 60,000 U.S. sterilizations—20,000 in California. North Carolina allowed sterilization of people with an IQ below 70—the bottom 3% of the intellectual population.

As we all know, purebred dogs, thoroughbred horses and every type of domesticated animal have been genetically improved. But faulty genes can also be passed on.

EU-PARENTING AND PARENT LICENSING

Looking deeper at the overpopulation, we should see that it is not enough to reduce the total population, if we want a peaceful, cooperative, contended, happy and productive world, we must attempt to reduce genetic diseases, reduce negative epigenetic changes (environmental stresses that may affect how genes function), and do what we can to insure that children are raised in a loving and emotionally nourishing environment.

There is a great deal of evidence that genetic tendencies, aroused or quieted by epigenetic and environmental factors are significantly related to both childhood and adult tendencies to abuse—from bullying to terrorism. So if we are to look at controlling the quantity of population, we should also look at improving the quality of the population by upgrading the quality of parenting.

There is no situation as pleasant and exciting as the frivolity that usually goes with the release of sperm that may impregnate an ovum and begin the process that eventually leads to birth, then death. But the simplicity of the start of impregnation does not signal the complicated consequences of the birth, education, and development of the child and adolescent that resulted from that moment of pleasure. So simple to start a life-- so difficult to develop a loving, healthy and educated young adult.

In order for the embryo and fetus to develop into a healthy baby requires the proper nutrition of the mother, competent medical attention, and a pregnancy which is as stress-free as is possible. We have known for many years that genetics are important, if not essential, for a healthy baby. For the last 30 years we have become aware that epigenetics (the science of environmental effects that can change the functions of the genes, making them active or inactive.

We now know that certain experiences of parents or other ancestors can be passed on to a child. Alcoholism, drug use or abuse, starvation or overeating, and to a large degree--stresses of various sorts, can inactivate genes that may be essential in the ability of the child to live fully. As safe as you may think life is in the placenta, research shows that stresses undergone by the mother can seriously affect the genes of the developing embryo or fetus. Stresses throughout life, especially early in life, can have significant effects on the development of a child and adolescent. These may be registered as epigenetic changes on the genes or as conscious or unconscious scars on the psyche.

Then there are the obvious needs of a child: nutrition, disease prevention, emotional warmth and love, education and a number of other factors that can positively or negatively affect the child or adolescent.

Raising a child is probably the most important job in the world. It requires a significant knowledge of nutrition, medicine, psychology, and educational attainment-- along with the relatively rare ability to love. We could also say that a certain amount of money will be needed to assure that the child has its physical needs met.

Barbers and cosmetologists, doctors and nurses, teachers and drivers-- all need licenses. They also all need training. What kind of training does a parent need? As indicated above, it should be extensive. Plus, we would need to be certain that the parents had the ability to love the child.

While a basic knowledge of nutrition and health may be easily obtained, understanding the psychological needs of the child is extremely complicated. So let us look for a few minutes at some of the needs of a child as it grows. We can see here why it would be so difficult to develop a license for parents. But we can also see why prospective parents should have such basic knowledges. If we were to require a knowledge of child psychology in order to have a child, probably many people would opt out-- and solve our population problem!

We will look for a few moments at what a few of the major world authorities on children and adults have to say. First we will summarize some of the thoughts of psychologists and educators such as Erik Erikson and Robert Havighurst. Then we will see what Erik Fromm has to say about psychological needs and how the ability to love develops. We will glance at what Abraham Maslow has to say about how our motivations. Then we will look at how Piaget and Kohlberg find how values are developed.

EU-PARENTING

A major question is whether or not children should have parents who can take care of them physically, emotionally, and educationally. Traditionally we have given the rights to adults to have children-- and to educate them the way they wish. We see both rich and poor adults who are highly competent as parents, and we see both rich and poor adults who are ineffective and often, highly destructive to their children. Some even murder them. Many abuse them severely both mentally and physically.

There is probably no activity more pleasant for the adults than the action of attempting to have the sperm meet a friendly ovum. From, there on there may be joys or pains through the period of pregnancy to childbirth.

After the birth, there is no job that requires the knowledge and the abilities to perform them as much as does parenthood. To be effective, it takes an incredible amount of the ability to love. It takes knowledge of the physical body, how it grows, and the physical and emotional needs of the child through the various stages of life. It requires a great deal of time. Many parents rationalize that they give quality time to their children since they don't have a great deal of the quantity of time to spend with them daily. In truth, children need both quantity and quality of time from their parents.

LICENSING PARENTS

What you find out in the United Nations Declaration of Human Rights is that it gives adults the right to "start a family." But it doesn't give the potential children the right to effective loving parenting. In fact, no rights for children begin until they are born.

We can't know if a child would prefer not to be born if he inherited physical diseases like hemophilia (inability of blood to clot), Down syndrome (severe learning disability), cystic fibrosis, Tay Sacks disease, sickle cell anemia, or any of the other genetic physical problems. Mental disorders may also be passed on genetically or epigenetically, such as: autism, attention deficit hyperactivity disorder (ADHD), bipolar disorder, major depression and schizophrenia.

Until recently, when the Israeli Supreme Court stopped the practice, children were suing their parents for "wrongful birth" because they wished they had never been born.

WRONGFUL BIRTH

In some jurisdictions, the child, sometimes with his or her parents, can sue the doctors or the hospital for not discovering a birth defect. California, India, The Netherlands (and previously Israel), have allowed for "wrongful life" actions when children are born with disabilities—or have lived unhappy lives.

In 2019, a businessman in Mumbai, India sued his lawyer parents saying that he should not have to suffer through life because of society's problems just because his parents wanted a few moments of pleasure.

"Wrongful life" or "wrongful birth" are the legal terms most commonly used where a child or the child's legal guardian sues the parents, the doctors, or the medical personnel involved in a birth that the offspring believes to be not in his or her interest. It may be because of faulty genetic testing, examinations during pregnancy, or being brought into a world that was not comfortable.

Such legal actions have been used in Israel by a number of disabled people who felt that their lives were miserable because of their birth. Some sued their parents. Some sued the medical profession. Parents also have been involved as plaintiffs against doctors or hospitals because they were not notified of potential genetic problems.

The Supreme Court of Israel has now made it illegal to sue for wrongful birth. The Supreme Court of California, however, has allowed it. In the 1982 case of Curlander v Bio-Science Laboratories, was a case in which the child was born with Tay-Sachs disease when the parents relied on the genetic testing of the laboratory and were not given the correct information, so did not proceed with amniocentesis. The Court's opinion included this paragraph:

"The reality of the 'wrongful-life' concept is that such a plaintiff both exists and suffers, due to the negligence of others. It is neither necessary, nor just, to retreat into meditation on the mysteries of life. We need not be concerned with the fact that had defendants not been negligent, the plaintiff might not have come into existence at all. The reality of genetic impairment is no longer a mystery. In addition, a reverent appreciation of life compels recognition that plaintiff, however impaired she may be, has come into existence as a living person with certain rights." (106 Cal Ap 3d 83)

The Curlander decision gives interested readers an extensive history of the cases in the U.S. that involve "wrongful life."

A similar case had a similar conclusion in New York, but it was overruled by the Supreme Court of New York. Many other states and countries have taken the same route, in disallowing wrongful birth actions. In Germany, the Federal Constitutional Court ruled that "the life of the disabled person is as valuable as a non-disabled person. because, human dignity is a basic concept in the German Constitution." But, the theoretical rationalization probably does not adequately comfort an unhappy, or miserable, living person. (As previously mentioned, our values can be based on self-centered assumptions, God-based assumptions, or society based assumptions. In this case, the complaining person was using self-centered assumptions, while the judges used a society-based, or possibly even a God-based, assumption. So we have the common conflict between value assumptions in our lives.)

(For those who would like to explore our values decision or the bases of our morality in depth, read "On Human Values," Book 4 of the free e-book series "And Gulliver Returns." The book is also available in print.)

In 2005, the Dutch Supreme Court upheld a lower court decision for a verdict for wrongful life.

Some courts have held that "nonexistent persons" do not have rights. This would of course indicate that life does not start until sometime after conception. In Israel, 600 cases for wrongful birth had been heard before the concept was made illegal.

In the Indian case the plaintiff's mother said that she "would destroy her son in court."

In the UK. a report by a cross-party committee found that almost one-in-five children under the age of 15 are growing up in a home that has "limited access to food ... due to lack of money or other resources." The 56-page report added. Yet, Britain is the world's fifth-richest country.

Then, we might look at the Preamble to the American Constitution, which sounds good but cannot be used in court. We will quote it again.

"We the people of the United States, in order to form a more perfect union, establish justice, insure domestic tranquility, provide for the common defense, promote the general welfare, and secure the blessings of liberty to ourselves and our posterity, do ordain and establish this Constitution for the United States of Amer ica."

We therefore might ask:

> Is it "just" to have babies born to parents who do n't want them?
> Is it "just" to have babies born to parents who smoke, knowing the harmful effects of passive smoke?
> Is it "just" to have children born to alcoholics or to addicts of other drugs?
> Is it "just" to have children born into poverty when they may be malnourished or deprived of an adequate education?

We can ask the same questions about whether an unwanted child, or a child without a maximum chance at being the best that he or she can be, promotes the general welfare.

Would the child have a happier and more productive life if he or she were not physically or mentally afflicted? Would the parents have a happier life raising a child without these genetic problems? Would society be better off if it did not have to spend money attempting to right the genetic wrongs?

WHAT ABILITIES DO EFFECTIVE PARENTS NEED?

It takes an incredible amount of ability to love. It takes knowledge of the physical and emotional needs of the child through the various stages of life. It requires a great deal of time. Many parents rationalize that they give quality time to the children since they don't have a great deal of the quantity of time to spend with them daily. In truth, children need both quantity and quality time from their parents.

Licensing parents to have children has been suggested by a number of public figures. Child psychologist, Dr. Jack Westman wrote a very interesting book on parent licensing. ("Licensing Parents" 1994) One of his considerations was that young people should not have children because they have not had enough experience with life to handle parenthood. They also usually did not have a sufficient amount of money to take care of the economic needs of the child.

Dr. Hugh LaFollette, a philosopher, has written that parents need to be licensed. He is currently the Cole Chair in Ethics at the University of South Florida. He teaches and writes in ethics, especially practical ethics. He is author of books on applied ethics, such as gun control, and he is Editor-in-Chief of the International Encyclopedia of Ethics. See his article in the Princeton University Press in 1980:
http://www.hughlafollette.com/papers/licensing.parents.pdf

The free e-book series, "And Gulliver Returns" looks at a number of obstacles to licensing parents and also at a number of requirements that psychologists and educators have considered important for a growing child. http://andgulliverreturns.info/

If drivers, barbers and plumbers must be licensed, is raising a child as important as driving a car, getting a haircut, or changing a water pipe? We require licenses for the pediatricians who might treat the child for illnesses. We require child dentists to have licenses, so that they can work effectively with the tooth fairy.

My nephew, who is an incredibly dedicated high school English teacher, and his wife, a licensed clinical social worker, wanted to adopt a black child. The adoption process took months of vetting them by the state of Nevada and cost them over $20,000 to become parents of an unwanted child. The birth parents were teenage Las Vegas high school students. These students didn't need to pay a fee, be thoroughly investigated, or have a license. The lucky child has two incredibly loving parents who are raising him in an unbelievably enriched environment.

But, I understand that there are some children born into this world who are starving. Others are physically and mentally abused. Still others are sex slaves. How sad!

WHO IS MORE IMPORTANT, THE CHILD, THE PARENTS, OR THE SOCIETY?

The needs of society are changing very rapidly. Throughout most of our human history, the economic needs were for hunters, herders, and farmers. More children were often an advantage. As our economic society developed we needed more trades-people and manufacturers. Now machines can do much of our work. But the machines require electrical energy. This often pollutes when it is generated. But we don't need as many people. The number of unemployed people in the world of working age is over 170 million. The world's unemployment rate is just under 8%. So, do we really need this many people? Then, there are the homeless—over a half million in the U.S. and more than a quarter million in the UK. 18 million Indian children live on the streets. Homelessness is not a new phenomenon—when I was in Calcutta 55 years ago on a government assignment, I was told that 3,000 people died on the street every day. Wouldn't it be nice to have a society in which all, or most, people were living in their own homes, were well-fed, and were productive and happy?

If we are to attempt to guarantee every child a physically nourishing and loving environment we could probably solve the population problem immediately. The problem is that adults are guaranteed the right to have children no matter how harmful they might be to them. Probably most of us would agree that every child should be born into a family that is not impoverished and that is physically and emotionally nourishing.

The World Health Organization tells us that one person in four is undernourished and that 45% of all deaths to children under five (3.1 million children annually) are related to malnourishment. One in four children is stunted from malnutrition one in six children (100 million) is underweight.

One in five children in rich countries are born into poverty: 38% in Mexico, about 19% in the US and the UK, in Israel it is nearly 35%. Even rich Norway and Denmark are in the 9 to 10% range. Every country has children born into poverty. 25% of people in India are living below of poverty line of $1.90 income per day.

The hopeful, but uninformed, people among us assume that every child will be loved and cared for effectively. Naturally, every parent loves his child! But what is love? LOVE

One of America's greatest social thinkers, Ashley Montague, was asked to write the chapter on love for the Encyclopedia of Mental Health. Before he could write about love, he had to define it.

We use the word "love" in so many ways that its meaning is generally confused.
- "I love pizza."
- "I love Mickey Mouse."
- "God loves me."
- "I love my wife."
- "I love my children."

We see here several meanings of the word "love." Generally we use it to say, "I approve of." Montague's definition was quite the opposite. He saw love as being unselfish and intelligently informed. Here is his definition:

"Love is the communication to another person, of one's deep involvement in that person's welfare, of one's profound interest in him as a person, demonstrated by acts that support, stimulate and contribute to the realization of that person's potential and to the fulfillment of their personality."

Is the alcoholic parent capable of loving? More than 10% of American children live in households with at least one alcoholic parent. What about the drug addicted parent? 3% live in households with a parent who is drug addicted. What about the parent who smokes? What about the parent who has no knowledge of nutrition? What about the parent who does not understand the psychological stages that children will probably pass through? What about the parent who wants the child for what the child can do for them, rather than what they can do for the child?

WHAT ARE THE PSYCHOLOGICAL AND EMOTIONAL NEEDS OF THE CHILD?

It is obvious that parents should have a thorough knowledge of nutrition and diet, a knowledge of communicable diseases and how to prevent them, a knowledge of the importance of physical fitness and safety, a knowledge of how to educate the child effectively, and a knowledge of the psychological and emotional needs of the child. And, at least as important, is the ability to use these knowledges with the unselfish ability to love— and sometimes, infinite patience.

Looking at all of these ideals, we might wonder if any adults are capable of being effective parents!! Oh well, "perfection" is seldom, if ever, achieved—but we can, at least, strive to be better. And, certainly, all children born into the world should be raised by loving parents. So whether our main goal is to reduce climate change or foster a more effective society—giving all babies a real chance for a happy and productive life should be high on the list of the intelligent citizens of the world.

Let us look for a few moments at the informed observations of some highly respected psychologists and educators: Erik Erikson, Robert Havighurst and Abraham Maslow. Both Eric Erickson and Robert Havighurst have spent considerable portions of their lives studying the needs of children and adolescents. You may be interested in reading their thoughts.

Havighurst looked at both the physical and mental tasks that we must accomplish at each age. Erikson looked at the deeper psychological needs we must master. And, Maslow looked at the physical, emotional and intellectual needs we must fulfil to become "truly human" people.

HAVIGHURST

Robert Havighurst emphasized that learning is essential and that it continues throughout the life span. Growth and development occurs in six stages. He called these "developmental tasks."

Developmental Tasks of Infancy and Early Childhood:
1. Learning to walk.
2. Learning to take solid foods
3. Learning to talk
4. Learning to control the elimination of body wastes
5. Learning sex differences and sexual modesty
6. Forming concepts and learning language to describe social and physical reality.
7. Getting ready to read

Middle Childhood:
1. Learning physical skills necessary for ordinary games.
2. Building wholesome attitudes toward oneself as a growing organism
3. Learning to get along with age-mates
4. Learning an appropriate masculine or feminine social role
5. Developing fundamental skills in reading, writing, and calculating
6. Developing concepts necessary for everyday living.
7. Developing conscience, morality, and a scale of values

8. Achieving personal independence

9. Developing attitudes toward social groups and institutions

ERIKSON

Erikson called the early years of life <u>the sensory stage.</u> During this time the infant is a passive receiver of messages bombarding its senses. It is at this time, while the infant is totally dependent on others, that the first crisis is met. The baby learns whether to *"trust or mistrust"* the environment. This stage occurs during the first year or year-and-a-half of life. With the pursuit of money, rather than effective child raising, so common at every class level and with the great number of one-parent families, infants may have little opportunity to successfully meet this stage.

Erikson believed that a second stage, called <u>the muscular development stage</u> was next. If the child learns to control its muscular development (such as crawling, walking, and its bladder and bowel functions) successfully. It begins to feel that it is able to control the environment in some way. Erikson called this autonomy. But if there is a failure to adequately master one's musculature the child will develop a feeling of shame and will doubt its ability to successfully confront the world. This crisis Erikson called *"autonomy vs. shame and doubt. "* This should occur between the ages one and three.

How well a child handles these tasks is a major determinant as to whether he or she will develop a good feeling of self esteem <u>or </u>have a significant inferiority complex. These first few years are absolutely critical. It is highly unlikely that these tasks can be successfully completed in a day-care center. It is a very strong argument for one of the parents to be with the child most of the time during the first four or five years. (Who said parenting was easy??)

<u>The locomotor control stage </u>is a third stage which Erikson sees for our early years. The child attempts to find its own way-- to assert its needs and gain its rewards. Another problem of this age is that the child is attracted to the parent of the opposite sex (in Freudian terms, the Oedipus or Electra complex) and is somewhat alienated by the parent of the same sex. If the child is able to successfully solve the problems according to the behaviors which society considers acceptable, the child can be said to have developed "initiative. "If not, the child develops a sense of guilt which may remain forever as a part of its psychological make-up. This is called the crisis of *"initiative vs. guilt."* This would probably occur about age four to five. With so many absent parents and one parent families, the child may have a difficult time meeting this need. The pursuit of money by so many parents may leave the children without the opportunity to solve this "crisis."

MIDDLE CHILDHOOD

HAVIGHURST

According to Havighurst, from ages 6 to 11 new tasks are required to be learned. The developing child needs to learn:

1. The physical skills necessary to play ordinary games (catching, throwing, kicking, swimming, handling simple tools),
2. To build wholesome attitudes toward oneself as a growing person,
3. To get along with others of the same age,
4. To perform the appropriate social roles to function in the society,
5. To use the basic intellectual tools such as reading, writing, mathematics,
6. To develop basic concepts necessary for everyday living, such as ideas about health, history, geography, time, space, goal setting,
7. To hold a value system and a set of morals to guide behavior,
8. To develop a sense of independence,
9. To develop democratic attitudes toward society.

While the parents have primary responsibility for the early years of development, both the parents and the school must take responsibility for these middle years of childhood. Many adults have not mastered all of these developmental tasks themselves. There are adults who are not independent. There are adults who do not subscribe to the democratic ethic. There are adults who cannot read or write or who do not understand the basic concepts of history, geography, or health.

ERIKSON AGAIN

Erikson saw a latent stage in our development. During this stage the child needs to become competent in dealing with the world. Success in school or games might develop a feeling of competence in the child. But failure to meet this crisis would result in a feeling of <u>inferiority and failure</u>. This is called the ***"industry vs. inferiority"*** crisis, and is likely to occur between ages six and eleven. This is another important step in developing self-esteem and eliminating or reducing inferiority feelings in the child.

Upper and middle class families are likely to put their children into sports, such as Little League, into dance lessons or music classes, or into Scout activities. Those in the lower social classes don't always have these opportunities. Their world may be limited to school and the streets around home.

EARLY ADOLESCENCE

According to Havighurst, from age 12 the child must learn to become more independent and to take care of himself or herself. At this age it is important to get along with others of the same age while developing appropriate social roles (often denoted as masculine or feminine). The child should be becoming more independent of parents while developing a moral-ethical system. It is also important to develop appropriate and wholesome attitudes toward the social groups and the institutions that make up the society.

Erikson saw this period of <u>puberty and adolescence </u>as requiring that the individual confront the crisis of "***identity vs. role confusion***." It is essential to determine how one will feel about one's sexuality. It is also important to develop a code of values and to make some decisions relative to what occupations one might pursue. The child must develop the idea that he or she is a special person--a special person who is responsible for himself or herself.

Many youth, particularly boys, get their "identity" through painting graffiti on walls. Many young girls get their identity by having sexual relations and becoming teenage mothers. Neither of these types of behaviors can be said to be "appropriate" in terms of developing a suitable self-concept.

LATER ADOLESCENCE

At this time in a person's life, the peer group usually becomes more important. It is essential to develop more mature relationships with age mates of both sexes. Sexual attraction becomes intensely important. The development of adult sex roles as masculine or feminine--understanding the expected roles of our culture as well as the potential roles which society is opening up-- is often more difficult to achieve. The traditional success oriented masculine role of provider is easier for boys to achieve than it is for girls. Even today girls often have to struggle to break the traditional nurturing role of wife-mother in order to satisfy their power drives in other areas, such as law, medicine, or business. But now, of course, most countries have more female students than males in the universities.

HAVIGHURST

The maturing adolescent must come to grips with the facts that he or she:
1. Possesses a body which must be cared for;
2. Needs to develop the intellectual skills and concepts necessary for civic competence;
3. Must soon become psychologically independent of parents;
4. Must develop the knowledge and skills necessary for economic independence;
5. Must select and prepare for an occupation;
6. Should prepare for marriage and family life, prepare to live independently, or prepare for an alternative companionate life style.

7. Should develop a socially acceptable philosophy of life (a set of ethical standards necessary to behave in a socially responsible manner).

The best thing you can do for your children is not a financial inheritance but rather good genes and a healthy early environment. Warren Buffet, one of the world's richest men implied something like this when he said "Leave children enough money so that they feel they can do anything, but not enough so they can do nothing."

Parents who agree on how to raise their children are more effective than those who do not agree. Less authoritarian upbringing seems best. (This doesn't mean letting them do what they want--but rather not telling them everything to do.)

All loving parents want to give their children whatever physical and emotional ingredients are necessary to make that child the best that it can be. In the 18 or so years that the child is under the parents' custody, the parents will be determining the physical, intellectual and emotional structure of the child. Many thousands of inputs will determine the body and character of the future adult. But where can the parent look for guidance? The myriad of books often confuse the baffled parent even more.

INTELLECTUAL DEVELOPMENT

Intellectual development can be affected by the genes a child inherits and by the nutrition received in the womb and during the first years after birth. Psychologists have estimated that 7 per cent of children are born sufficiently defective so that their learning ability is impaired.

Whatever an infant's potential at the time of birth, it can be aided or frustrated by the environment in which it lives. The critical period in an infant's intellectual development begins at the age of seven months. By the age of three years, the child has usually mastered the beginnings of language which will be used in conversation throughout life, the adaptation to the role in the family, and many of the adjustment patterns which will be used during its lifetime. If the child is significantly behind others of the same age in these skills, it may be difficult to catch up. By the age of 4 approximately 50 per cent of the individual's intellectual development has taken place.

By eight years of age, approximately 80 per cent of the intellectual development has occurred.

Reading is the fundamental skill necessary to intellectual development. If a parent wants the child to learn to read, the best thing is to hold that child on one's lap and read stories aloud--over and over again, if necessary. The printed page, a reassuring voice, a fascinating story, and the physical comfort all indicate to the child that reading is a great source of pleasure. Cuddling is almost as important as the story in developing this idea. Of course, you can always buy a smart phone and let it raise your kids!

The United States Air Force recently compiled a list of indicators which may help to identify potential academic failure. Over-indulgent parents lead the list. A child should not be given all that he or she desires. The lessons of discipline and the rewards of work must be learned. Parents who coerce the child into studying can develop resentment against both the parents and the joy of learning.

Another factor leading to academic failure is starting the child to school too early. Just because a child is six-years-old does not mean that it is time to be in the first grade. People mature at different rates. Early academic failures may never be overcome. Unhappily, many parents are ashamed if their children are not "in the proper grade." But it is what is best for the child that should be considered to be primary. Other factors identified by the Air Force which were related to academic problems were: speech disorders, alcoholic parents, and premature birth.

VALUE DEVELOPMENT

Value development, like other areas of our development, is learned best by being rewarded for proper behavior rather than being punished for improper behavior, although either can be effective. We learn our values better by imitating our parents than by being told what to do.

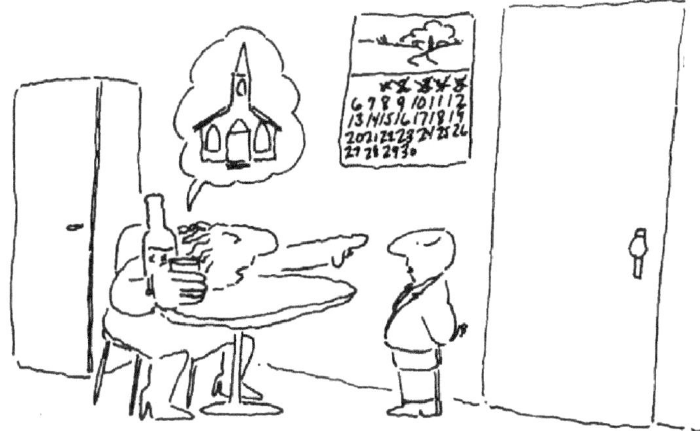

All parents should remember that some day their children will follow their example, rather than their advice.

In every area of life, we have developed value standards. How fast we drive, how much we pay for food, and whether we cheat on tests, are all values that we have learned. Many of these are the result of parental influence. If you wish your children to develop certain values, you will need to develop an atmosphere of both freedom and limitation. That may sound incongruous, but the limitations put on a child often allow more freedom by giving the child mental boundaries and security.

Television has a great impact on the values of most of the children who watch it. It teaches them to cope with frustration through violence, develops their taste in cereals, and determines their lists for Santa Claus. The average first grader has watched 5,000 hours of TV and the average high-school graduate has spent 11,000 hours in class but 19,000 hours watching television, during which time 200,000 violent acts and 40,000 murders have been witnessed. It might be assumed that many of the young adults' values have been infused by the "tube." Other countries do not allow the violence to be shown on television but then their constitutions do not allow the often harmful "freedom of speech" that American entertainment corporations enjoy. And, they don't have the number of mass shootings of today's American wild west.

Television viewing is being somewhat reduced as social media and gaming take up our recreational time. The average teen-age girl spends over 9 hours a week gaming, boys spend over 16 hours. The average person spends slightly over an hour a day on social media—up from twenty minutes seven years ago. We are certainly being entertained, but are we spending much time constructively developing ourselves or our society--or the children we are raising?

It appears that making money is far more important to America than raising non-violent highly valued children. Of course, the movie and television industries might not have enough imaginative minds to create programs like Madam Secretary or Mash. It doesn't take a great deal of imagination to write a script with a car chase or have twenty people cut up with a chain saw or shot with an assault weapon.

The Scientific Advisory Committee to the Surgeon General reported that there is a causative relationship between televised violence and later anti-social behavior in many cases. The committee said very young children cannot distinguish between fantasy and reality on TV; the children also see each incident in a story as a whole, unrelated to the total story (i.e., they don't realize that the robber was caught and imprisoned for his crime--the crime and the capture are often unrelated in the child's mind). The report found that children spend more time watching adult shows than children's programs. And, because television is "sanitized, " the children do not see all of the facts such as, the mutilated body of the victim of a crime or accident, or the sorrow of a family which has been broken by the murder of one of its members.

Television can increase the child's vocabulary in early years. However, children who continue to watch television constantly during the teen-age years have been found to be less bright than the occasional viewers.

MORALS AND VALUES

The leading theorists of the psychology of morals are probably the Swiss psychologist Jean Piaget and the Harvard psychologist Lawrence Kohlberg. Dr. Kohlberg has identified six levels of moral behavior.

The first two levels of learning how to behave in an ethical way are called "pre-moral" and are typical of children and juvenile delinquents. Stage one is the obedience of the child through the fear of punishment. Stage two is called reciprocity. The child will do something good if rewarded. The reward should be tangible, like candy, money, or praise.

The second two levels are called "conventional" morality. Kohlberg believes that most teenagers and adults work at this level most of the time. Stage three is the level in which people do good in order to be looked upon with the esteem of others. During adolescence, the esteem may come primarily from the peer group rather than the family. Stage four occurs when people's behavior and their ideas of right and wrong are developed; they believe that, in order for society or a group to function, one must obey authority, such as the law.

The last two levels of behavior are based on "principle. " Stage five is based on the people working within a framework of rules upon which they have mutually agreed. This happens when people believe in the Constitution because they feel that the ideas were developed to protect individual liberties and rights. Only about 1 adult in 4 works at this level. The sixth level deals with universal principles. These moral principles are considered to be applicable to all human beings and are so important that one would give up one's life for one's principles. Very few people work at this level. Perhaps Mahatma Gandhi or Martin Luther King would be recent examples of such principled people.

Parents often try to teach values by preaching, but this isn't usually too effective. The father who advises against smoking while opening his second pack of cigarettes is not likely to be believed. Parents who realize the importance of the values that they are demonstrating for their children often reevaluate them. Parents cannot help but teach values. They may teach drunkenness, speeding, violence, or they may teach honesty, loyalty, and justice. It is a very important undertaking, deserving of some deep and honest thought. But whoever said that raising children was easy?

As indicated earlier, I am against most youth sports which are organized by adults. When children and adolescents organize their own games they make certain that the rules are enforced. In basketball they may say "Call your own fouls." Playing touch football in the streets the teen-agers won't tolerate unfair play and will exclude those who don't play fair. These children are working at the fourth and fifth levels of moral development (the development of right and wrong and working together with mutually formulated behaviors). But when parents come into the picture and referees are hired to "find" the illegal behavior and to penalize the guilty culprits, the players are back to level one (fear of punishment).

(Please don't read the foregoing as an anti-sport statement but rather as a pro-child statement. As one who has taught physical education for 40 years, is a lifetime member of the American Football Coaches Association and has coached football for over 40 years, I am definitely for sport. But not for the professionalization or *parentization* of children's play and sport. Sport is probably the best vehicle to teach values that has ever been developed. But just as a poor English teacher can prejudice a child against our great language and literature, and a poor history teacher can kill a student's interest in developing the absolutely essential knowledge of our human heritage, a poor coach can eliminate the essential values lessons that sport can teach better than any other aspect of our education system.)

EMOTIONAL DEVELOPMENT

Emotional development is enhanced by many of the areas previously covered.

Cuddling the child while feeding it or reading to it, demonstrating stable values which give the child a sense of security, and giving time to the child in the day to day activities-- all have positive effects on the emotional health of the child.

When children do not feel the security or self-respect necessary for their emotional well-being, which parents should give, there is a good chance that the child will show the effects. Juvenile delinquency, harmful drug use, failure in school, poor social development, and even early marriage can be traced to unfulfilled emotional needs. The increase in stresses, the conflicts of values, and the less personal, more automated society are held responsible for the 65 per cent increase of children being treated in mental health facilities. The same factors may be partially responsible for the high rate of suicide in the fifteen to twenty-four-year-age group. The fact that one in nine youths under nineteen has appeared before a juvenile court is also an indication of the values children hold. Somewhere along the line, the society, particularly some parents, have failed miserably in developing the emotional stability of their children.

In more primitive societies, the communities generally take more responsibility for the raising of children. But in our society the brunt of the load falls on the parents to do this enormous job. Because so many parents fail, we can certainly say that, in general, in the United States our children may be our most neglected citizens.

Most parents are quite content to change diapers for a few weeks and to show off the new baby to their friends and relatives. And most parents find many joys aiding in the development of their children. But a great many new parents seem to be counting the days until the child will be in a full-time nursery school, and the parent will be freed of the responsibility of raising the child. Recently there has been a great outcry, particularly from the feminist groups, to have publicly-paid child care centers available, so that mothers can get back into the work force where they are happier. This simple solution may relieve a parent of "feeling tied down," but there is a great deal of evidence to indicate that it may make the child feel "thrown out." It depends on the attentiveness of the care-givers at the school.

Reports from eastern Europe and the Soviet Union, before their freedom from the Communist regimes, indicated that children raised in full-time child-care centers had higher incidences of emotional disturbances, difficulties in school, and juvenile delinquency when compared with those children who had been raised at home. It appears that the problems were most pronounced among those who spent their earlier years (before they were five) in the centers.

It seems clear that if a couple wants children, there is a great need to be committed to them. It doesn't matter whether it is the mother or the father who stays home, but there must be somebody if the child is to have the best chance to feel wanted by his or her family and to be effectively socialized into that family. Having both parents in the home gives children a feeling of security and gives the children an idea of the ways a marriage can work and what roles can be played to make for a successful relationship.

There are millions of children living in broken homes. And there are millions of others who are living in families where the parents apparently don't care. Both parents may be working, be involved in outside activities, or doing so many other things that keep parents busy, busy, busy. So children can lose their parents by lack of concern as well as by divorce or death.

PSYCHOLOGICAL PARENTHOOD

Psychological parenthood is what children need. Many people assume that because two people were biologically capable of having a child, they are psychologically capable of caring for that child. But being able to perform sexual intercourse and being fertile enough to conceive a child are capabilities quite common in our species. The quality of emotional stability or the capacity to love and nurture a child, which are essential for effective parenting, are often lacking in the biological parents. Quite often too, people with the emotional abilities to be parents are sterile.

Some adult, preferably a parent, must take over the emotional development of the child. Usually this duty falls on the mother because: her hormones seem to make her more gentle; her nine months of pregnancy may give her a greater feeling of responsibility, the father is often the better income producer; and tradition has accepted the female in the "mothering" role. But in many cases men are far more competent than many women to raise their children.

Unhappily, many fathers and mothers will both abandon their duties of child raising. Sometimes it is ignorance of the needs of the child, other times it is the result of the adult being selfish. If the parents refuse to be responsible, most states have laws that can protect the child. The child can be placed with other relatives, in a foster home, or put up for adoption. But such actions are seldom taken unless the parents request it.

Many parents assume that they love their children simply because they provide for them. Nearly every animal also does this. The question is how much are we helping our children to grow independently so that they will be full-functioning adults. Since young children see the world through the lens presented by the experiences they have with their parents, it is essential that those experiences give the child the feeling of self-respect, love, and self-esteem that are necessary to function as emotionally mature adults. We know that such deprivation will have an effect on the emotional development of the child. But now there is evidence that such emotional losses may also show in stunted physical and intellectual growth. (There is evidence that the growth hormones are inhibited by a lack of parental love.)

The emotional needs of children are difficult to judge. Just as their rates of physical and intellectual growth are not exact, neither is their development of emotional maturity. Infants start life as selfish, helpless, asocial, emotional beings. The job of the parents, and later the schools, is to bring these non-socialized insecure infants to a point where they are loving, independent, social, and intellectual. We can see several paths of development of which parents should be aware.

THE PATHS OF EMOTIONAL GROWTH

Growing from selfishness to love is one of the primary goals of emotional development. If the child is cared for and comes to realize that people care, self-respect will develop. From this basis of self-respect, the ability to love will grow. Of course, obstacles can develop along the way. Jealousy of the child toward the parent of the opposite sex (the Oedipus complex) is not uncommon during the first few years of life. The child's love of, or rather need for, the other parent is threatened. The child's selfish desire for the parent will normally be overcome as the ability to love is developed. Parents can aid the children's development of the ability to love by encouraging them to show concern for others, such as writing a thank-you note to Aunt Ann, giving to United Way, or baby-sitting for friends.

Erich Fromm wrote one of the classic books on love (The Art of Loving). He said that "we learn to love by being loved." He then suggested an evolution of the ability to love.

> Self love—the singular concern with self, which is the domain of infants;
> Recognition that others are also "selfs."
> Ability to be greatly concerned with (to be able to love unselfishly) one or a few others.
> The generalized ability to love—humanitarian love. We often see this recognized in Nobel Peace Prize winners, like Mother Theresa, Albert Schweitzer, and Bishop Tutu.

The evolution from helplessness to independence is a second path of emotional growth. The child will be taught to drink from a cup, keep the bedroom neat, and do chores around the house. Parents should begin to allow children to make decisions as they become intellectually ready. At first, it may be, "Do you want vanilla or chocolate ice cream?" Later it might be, "Do you want to go with us or stay at home?" or "Do you plan on taking Spanish or German?" As the child learns to take responsibility, more independent thinking may develop.

Models will often be selected as exhibiting life styles that will allow the child to make decisions about particular goals. Early in life the goal of being a cowboy or a firefighter may predominate. Later it may be a sports idol or an entertainment figure. If these are seen to be unachievable, the older child will probably look towards occupational fields which arc compatiblc with its developing interests and academic aptitudes.

A third pattern of emotional growth is found in **the asocial to social progression**. The infant has no social concept. Soon a relationship will be developed with one or both parents. Next it is normal to learn to play alone while sitting near another child who is also playing alone. The next stage of social growth is playing together with a friend of the same sex, then a group of friends of the same sex. Generally by age eight, groups of children will play together. Larger groups of the same sex (gangs or clubs) may develop in the teenage years. In the early teenage years, an interest in sexual relationships develops. The eventual goal of this path of development is to be at ease with all people. With this end in view, parents should not only attempt to expose their children to the appropriate groups of children, but should also be aware of their need to be able to be at ease with adults. Parents who hide their children from adult company, telling them to "go downstairs and watch the TV, " may not be doing the most they can to aid in the child's socialization. Without adequate socialization, the child will probably be introverted and lacking in a feeling of adequacy in this area.

A fourth area of concern is the **emotional to intellectual continuum.** A newborn child has only emotions. It can express fear and a few other reactions which are not unlike animals. But the child has the potential to become a being able to make decisions based on evidence. The human brain is uniquely capable of acquiring facts and feelings that can then be viewed from a variety of perspectives and can form the evidence from which decisions are made. In order to make the child's mind ready to assimilate knowledge the child will have to learn to listen, to speak, to read, and to count. Making decisions which are based on the best evidence (the scientific method) is one of the important skills to be mastered in this area of development.

This is not an all-inclusive list of emotional tasks which the child on the path to mature adulthood must master. These broad goals can be further divided. For example, we could look at the broad range of activities from the simplest to the complex. We could explore "learning to count to learning advanced calculus" or a "learning the alphabet to writing a book." But it would take several more books to expand on the possibilities.

These different experiences which a child may be given are not totally independent. For example, developing physical skills such as drinking from a cup, walking, riding a bicycle, and serving a tennis ball are useful in developing independence and becoming more social. Learning to read could help in any of the above-mentioned areas.

You can also see that each of these areas of development may never be achieved by any one person. If Fromm is right and the ultimate ability in loving is when a person can love the whole human race, then that ultimate ability to love is seldom realized. If the objective of intellectual competence includes the ability to look objectively at the evidence and make the best decision and to become fully self-actualized people, this too is seldom achieved. It is not necessary that the parents successfully guide their children along each of these paths, only that they start them and guide them an appropriate distance for each age level.

If a child needs help in reading, the parent should provide that help. If a child needs more socialization experiences, the parent should provide the setting. If a child is not making strides toward independence, the parent should aid in that direction. Since there are no absolute guidelines as to what should be done each month for each child, the parent is left to his or her own devices. The concerned parent can look at the evidence available, then do the best job possible--realizing that there has probably never been a perfect parent. *"Thank goodness! For a while it looked like the pressure was really on, didn't it?"*

There will be apparent failures along the way. Your four-year-old may become quite stubborn and maybe throw a temper tantrum. Don't worry, it's all part of the "becoming independent" path. And when your 13-year-old would rather go camping with friends than go to Hawaii with you, she's just showing some independence. And that's what you want as a parent. But if your 16-year-old elopes with the plumber, there may be a problem, because eloping is not the best method of showing independence.

MASLOW'S HIERERARCHY OF MOTIVATION

Abraham Maslow began his life as a behaviorist psychologist. As he matured, however, he became a humanist--thinking that humans are quite different from others in the animal kingdom. He looked at us as having several levels of motivations. As we satisfy one level we are ready to go to the next stage in humanness. Many of the ideas of others, like Freud's idea of sexuality, and Adler's idea that we have a need for power over ourselves and our world, can be found at different levels of Maslow's 'hierarchy of needs.'

Maslow wrote that the most basic drives are physiological. If we are not satisfied, our whole being pursues them. For example, if I am very hungry or very thirsty the desire to satisfy these basic needs will take precedence over any other desires I might have. Once these most basic needs are met my next need is safety. If I feel physically and emotionally safe I then would want love. If I am loved, the next most important need is esteem, such as the recognition of others. I can then pursue the highest human needs, those of 'self-actualization.' These needs Maslow called the *meta* needs. '*Meta*' is from the Greek word meaning 'highest.'

SELF-ACTUALIZATION (Meta needs--Morality, creativity, spontaneity, problem solving, lack of prejudice, acceptance of facts).

^

ESTEEM (Belonging, Self-esteem, confidence, achievement, respect of others, respect by others.)

^

LOVE (Friendship, family, intimacy.)

^

SAFETY (Security of body, of employment, of resources, of morality, of the family, of health, of property.)

^

PHYSIOLOGICAL (Breathing, food, water, sex, sleep, homeostasis, excretion)

The physiological need for air is accomplished without even thinking about it. We don't have to say to ourselves 'inhale, exhale.' It is done unconsciously. Hunger pangs develop unconsciously but our conscious mind picks up the signal and says, 'I'm hungry.' The erection of the penis or the lubrication of the vulva occur unconsciously, usually after the conscious mind says 'I want to make love.' We can see some similarities with Freud's ideas here.

The need for safety comes next up the hierarchy. If Tarzan has satisfied his needs for food and water he may build a tree house for his safety. However, if he is very hungry he may swim across a crocodile infested river to harvest a banana tree. An infant may seek the security of a parent's arms when encountering a threatening situation. A driver may buckle the shoulder strap because there is always the possibility of an auto accident.

I have heard that 80% of Italian men from 18 to 30 still live with their parents. I guess there is a lot of safety and security in having mama take care of you. When do they start becoming responsible for themselves and the society? Italy's tight society and strong family security run counter to the competitiveness needed in global economics. No need to fight dragons when you are safe in your castle.

Maslow's third step to mental health is the need for love and affection that can be met in the family, peer group, or in some other group in which emotional bonds are formed. The love need is aided by deep emotional ties. Maslow agrees with Fromm in his belief that a lack of love is the most commonly found reason for psychological maladjustment.

Moving to the next level we find the esteem needs that relate to a person's feelings of self-worth. If a person has been loved, it goes a long way towards helping to develop a feeling of self-respect. If a person obtains the respect and praise of other people, especially when young, there is a good chance of developing an adequate feeling of self-worth. We can see some of Adler's ideas here.

The physiological, safety, love and esteem needs are called 'basic needs' by Maslow. These needs should be easily met in any civilized society. Sadly, the love and esteem needs are not met as often as would be desirable. But if these 'basic needs' are met the individual can go on to satisfy the 'truly human needs' or as Maslow called them the 'meta needs.'

The meta needs include beauty, order, unity, justice, and goodness. When you successfully meet these needs you are 'self actualizing' or realizing your highest self. In his later work Maslow preferred the term becoming 'fully human' to the term 'self actualization' which he had used earlier.

While many psychologists have looked at mental illness-- then developed their theories of what mental health should be—the opposite of mental illness. Or rather, a life without the symptoms of a mental illness. (At that time, psychologists were not as aware of the genetic and epigenetic causes of the symptoms of mental illness,)

Maslow started by looking at mentally healthy people. He determined which people seemed to have their highest potentials realized, then he analyzed why they were healthy. These ideas about some people achieving at a 'truly human' level were initiated when Maslow decided to analyze two of his teachers. These two people held special places in his life. They were different. They were emotionally healthy. They were creative, happy and dynamic. After analyzing their characteristics, he began to look at other people who exhibited the highest human traits.

We can also learn much from self-actualizing, mentally healthy people. 'They have higher ceilings. They can see further. And they can see in a more inclusive and integrating way. They teach us that there is no real opposition between caution and courage, between action and contemplation, between vigor and speculation, between seriousness and high level humor ... such people feel no need to deny their deeper feelings. Indeed, it is my impression that, if anything, they tend to enjoy such experiences.

You can guess that developing children who are 'truly human' is a tall order for parents. We certainly don't expect every parent to raise a truly self-actualized child, but it should be a goal. We should give every assistance possible for this to happen—and it happens more than you might imagine.

Are any of these ideas important—or even essential, for parents in today's world?

CHILD ABUSE

Child abuse is, unhappily, a common phenomenon. It is a crime which is seldom reported. The estimates of actual cases are as high as 4,000,000 annually. Deaths from child abuse may number as many as 2,000 in the U.S. Usually the mother is the person guilty of beating the child. The father is likely to stand by, doing nothing. When parents of obviously battered children are confronted with the evidence, they are likely to say *"He fell out of the highchair,"* or *"I was giving her a bath and the phone rang; she drowned in the minute I was gone."* Usually the bruises on the child's body belie the parents' alibis. Sometimes the injuries and deaths are the results of a sudden uncontrollable frustration, other times they appear to be calculated cruelty and torture.

One recent case in California found that a mother and stepfather had made a four-year-old girl run around the house without stopping for two days until she died of exhaustion and from the beatings she received if she stopped running. The parents had previously served two years in jail for child abuse.

Child-abusing parents are likely to be mentally ill, alcoholics, or drug addicts. They are usually under twenty-five, but contrary to popular opinion, they may be at any economic, social, or intellectual level. They generally come from families in which they were beaten as children.

Generally child-beating parents are unable to cope with the problems of parenthood, especially a child's crying. A normal parent will most likely search for the cause of the child's crying, seeking outside help if necessary. The child abuser is more likely to yell at the child to "stop crying" even if the child is only a few months old. They also are likely to expect too much from a child. They may begin disciplining when the child is only three or four-months-old and may begin toilet training at six to eight months, long before the child is physiologically ready to be trained.

Nearly all parents are pushed beyond their endurance at some time. Nearly all parents will find it necessary to spank their children at some time. Both are normal. But if the parent loses control and the spanking becomes a beating, both the parent and the child become losers. The beaten child is a likely candidate for becoming maladjusted and eventually may behave as he or she has been treated--and another child beater is developed.

Now that society has recognized the extent and the severity of the problem, laws are being passed to require teachers and doctors to report incidents of abuse. Counseling centers are being expanded. Self-help groups, such as Parents Anonymous, are springing up all over the country. If you have been beaten as a child, it is quite possible that you might become a child abuser. You might well consider counseling before marriage, and you should give some consideration and study to the idea of being an effective parent.

Sexual abuse of children. We find sexual abuse in every area of life. Parents, stepparents, teachers, coaches, neighbors and others are often found to be sexual predators and abusers. We now find that in other parts of the world, parents are often selling their children into slavery and prostitution. Men are traveling to distant countries to have paid sex with children. Some children are forced into sexual situations then are videoed and exposed to the world. As caring parents we must guard against such actions against our own children and to work to prevent it with other children.

AND SO

Is this what we want for our children—abuse, neglect, experiencing hate?? Can parent licensing reduce this scourge while reducing the population and reducing warming? We know that it will probably never happen—BUT IT SHOULD! How important is our survival? How important are our children?

CHAPTER 12
ONWARD!

If it's true, like Toynbee said, that 'civilizations don't have to die—because they are not organisms, but rather products of wills'—then we have a chance.

– But the civilizations that he studied died. his life mission was to study 'why.'

But no civilization of the past has faced the threat that our whole species faces today. Maybe a few can realize that many people are living beyond the means that the planet can suppo, but can enough of the world's population see it, believe it, and start to do the drastic things needed to make it happen?

> ➤ Nature won't clear up the mess we have caused. **We** have to do it. We must find ways to reduce the greenhouse gases we produce and somehow store those we have produced.
> ➤ I think you guys should do it. I still want my Humvee which gets 6 miles to the gallon. I want speed and power.
> ➤ I want air conditioning in my twelve room house and in my car.

The realities are that most people don't want to sacrifice. Just look at the American personal debt. The average Americans not only want to have everything he or she already has, they want every one of the latest gadgets, cars, video games, and home appliances that is advertised. And they want it now!

They want the homes they can't afford—and the second home they can't afford. They want the boat they can't afford and the vacation they can't afford. There are so many living in a plastic card dream world—and it usually becomes a nightmare. Do you think that these people are willing to sacrifice anything? No matter how minor?

It's a self-centered morality that generally predominates over what's good for society or even what's good for themselves in the future. Eat, drink and be merry, for tomorrow we die—or go bankrupt. Look at the number of bankruptcies and home mortgage foreclosures of a few years ago. Home owners couldn't make their house payments. The mortgage lenders went bankrupt. The stock market dropped. Everything financially is inter-related. Our planet is in a worse condition than the home mortgage lenders. But the world can't declare bankruptcy. Either we live or we die. We won't get a second chance like an over-mortgaged home owner has.

But it depends on such things as the number of trees and other plants in the world and how much more CO_2 the ocean can absorb. It has been absorbing about half of the human produced CO_2 up to now. But as the ocean warms the CO_2 is held closer to the surface and the amount of gas that can be absorbed by the whole ocean is reduced.

Then there is the fact that when the climate warms, the plants don't absorb as much carbon dioxide, probably because they reduce their growing rate so that they can conserve water. So, CO_2 emissions are not being handled as well as they were a hundred years ago. But there's more to the mix. As the world warms, there is some evidence that the tree line is rising in the northern latitudes and in the higher altitudes. But then there are some other negatives like tree damaging insects that increase as the climate warms. The average temperature is expected to increase by almost one and a half degrees Celsius by 2050. It may not sound like much but on a global scale it is immense. If we do nothing, the Earth's temperature will probably rise 4 degrees Celsius this century.

Shall we work to stop it?

ARE WE UP TO THE CHALLENGE?

Index

N

O

P

Q

Qatar, 41

R

Rain, 5, 8–9, 15, 22, 26, 28, 31, 36, 40, 57

Retirement, 6–7, 54, 71, 74

Rhine, 29

Rice, 24, 39, 58

Russian Federation, 41

S

Sahara, 15, 27

Saudi Arabia, 41, 76

Self-centered values, 5, 44

Shells, 21

Sinks, 6, 9, 23, 66, 69

Skeptics, 4, 10, 12, 34

Snow, 8, 28, 36, 57, 62

Socialism, 78

Societal changes, 57–58

Society-based values, 5, 44

Solar, 25, 27, 30, 32, 42, 47, 55–56, 58–59, 61–62, 66, 68

Solar panels, 55, 58, 66

Solutions, 2, 6, 9, 13, 30, 33, 55, 57–58, 60–62

South Korea, 41

Southern Europe, 15–16, 26

Spain, 16, 23, 41

STEM graduates, 73

Storms, 4, 8, 15, 18, 22–23, 26, 28–29, 47, 57, 75, 77, 80

Sulfur dioxide, 22, 40

sustainable population, 70

T

Taxes, 6–7, 26, 29, 42, 48, 51–52, 61–62, 65, 68, 75, 77–78, 81, 83

Technology, 8–9, 72

television, 35, 52, 67–68, 77, 93–94

Tides, 4, 18–19

tradition, 3, 6, 26, 58, 70–71, 73–75, 77–78, 80, 96

Trees, 6, 12, 23, 30, 32–33, 42, 58–59, 61, 63, 66, 69, 71, 75–76, 102

Typhoons, 28

www.ingramcontent.com/pod-product-compliance
Lightning Source LLC
Chambersburg PA
CBHW081440250726
48662CB00009B/2885